Progress in Inflammation Research

Series Editor

Prof. Dr. Michael J. Parnham
PLIVA
Research Institute
Prilaz baruna Filipovica 25
10000 Zagreb
Croatia

Published titles:
T Cells in Arthritis, P. Miossec, W. van den Berg, G. Firestein (Editors), 1998
Chemokines and Skin, E. Kownatzki, J. Norgauer (Editors), 1998
Medicinal Fatty Acids, J. Kremer (Editor), 1998
Inducible Enzymes in the Inflammatory Response, D.A. Willoughby, A. Tomlinson (Editors), 1999
Cytokines in Severe Sepsis and Septic Shock, H. Redl, G. Schlag (Editors), 1999
Fatty Acids and Inflammatory Skin Diseases, J.-M. Schröder (Editor), 1999
Immunomodulatory Agents from Plants, H. Wagner (Editor), 1999
Cytokines and Pain, L. Watkins, S. Maier (Editors), 1999
In Vivo *Models of Inflammation*, D. Morgan, L. Marshall (Editors), 1999
Pain and Neurogenic Inflammation, S.D. Brain, P. Moore (Editors), 1999
Anti-Inflammatory Drugs in Asthma, A.P. Sampson, M.K. Church (Editors), 1999
Novel Inhibitors of Leukotrienes, G. Folco, B. Samuelsson, R.C. Murphy (Editors), 1999
Vascular Adhesion Molecules and Inflammation, J.D. Pearson (Editor), 1999
Metalloproteinases as Targets for Anti-Inflammatory Drugs, K.M.K. Bottomley, D. Bradshaw, J.S. Nixon (Editors), 1999
Free Radicals and Inflammation, P.G. Winyard, D.R. Blake, C.H. Evans (Editors), 1999
Gene Therapy in Inflammatory Diseases, C.H. Evans, P. Robbins (Editors), 2000
New Cytokines as Potential Drugs, S.K. Narula, R. Coffmann (Editors), 2000
High Throughput Screening for Novel Anti-Inflammatories, M. Kahn (Editor), 2000
Immunology and Drug Therapy of Atopic Skin Diseases, C.A.F.M. Bruijnzeel-Komen, E.F. Knol (Editors), 2000

Forthcoming titles:
Novel Cytokine Inhibitors, G.A. Higgs and B. Henderson (Editors), 2000
Cellular Mechanisms in Airway Inflammation, C. Page, K. Banner, D. Spina (Editors), 2000

Inflammatory Processes: Molecular Mechanisms and Therapeutic Opportunities

L. Gordon Letts
Douglas W. Morgan

Editors

Springer Basel AG

Editors

Dr. L. Gordon Letts
NitroMed Inc.
12 Oak Park Drive
Bedford, MA 01730
USA

Dr. Douglas W. Morgan
Abbott Laboratories
100 Abbott Park Road
Abbott Park, IL 60064
USA

Deutsche Bibliothek Cataloging-in-Publication Data

Inflammatory Processes : Molecular Mechanisms and Therapeutic Opportunities /
ed. by L.G. Letts , D.W. Morgan - Basel ; Boston ; Berlin : Birkhäuser, 2000
   (Progress in inflammation research)

ISBN 978-3-0348-9580-4   ISBN 978-3-0348-8468-6 (eBook)
DOI 10.1007/978-3-0348-8468-6

Originally published by Birkhäuser Verlag, Basel, Switzerland in 2000

Printed on acid-free paper produced from chlorine-free pulp. TCF ∞
Cover design: Markus Etterich, Basel
Cover illustration: Pathways leading to the activation of NF-κB (see page 24)

9 8 7 6 5 4 3 2 1

Contents

List of contributors

Robert T. Abraham, Department of Pharmacology and Cancer Biology, Room C333B LSRC, Box 3813, DUMC, Durham, NC 27710, USA; e-mail: abrah008@mc.duke.edu

Catherine Adams Burton, DuPont Pharmaceuticals Company, 500 S. Ridgeway Avenue, G-205 Glenolden, PA 19036, USA

Lisa A. Beck, Johns Hopkins University School of Medicine, Asthma and Allergy Center, 5501 Hopkins Bayview Circle, Baltimore, MD 21224, USA

Pamela Benfield, DuPont Pharmaceuticals Company, 500 S. Ridgeway Avenue, G-205 Glenolden, PA 19036, USA

John Boylan, DuPont Pharmaceuticals Company, Research and Development Experimental Station, P.O. Box 80400, Wilmington, DE 19880-0440, USA; has since moved to Amgen Inc., Thousand Oaks, California, USA

Marie Chabot-Fletcher, Department of Immunology, UW2531, SmithKline Beecham Pharmaceuticals, 709 Swedeland Rd., P.O. Box 1539, King of Prussia, PA 19406, USA; e-mail: marie_c_chabot-fletcher@sbphrd.com

Stephen W. Chensue, Department of Pathology, University of Michigan Medical School, 5214, Med Sci I, 1301 Catherine Road, Ann Arbor, MI 48109-0602, USA

Roger J. Davis, Howard Hughes Medical Institute, Program in Molecular Medicine, Department of Biochemistry and Molecular Biology, University of Massachusetts Medical School, 373 Plantation Street, Worcester, MA 01605, USA; e-mail: roger.davis@umassmed.edu

Long Gu, Department of Adult Oncology, Dana-Farber Cancer Institute, Harvard Medical School, 44 Binney Street, Boston, MA 02115, USA

Cory Hogaboam, Department of Pathology, University of Michigan Medical School, 5214, Med Sci I, 1301 Catherine Road, Ann Arbor, MI 48109-0602, USA

Janet Kerr, DuPont Pharmaceuticals Company, Research and Development Experimental Station, P.O. Box 80400, Wilmington, DE 19880-0440, USA

Steven L Kunkel, Department of Pathology, University of Michigan Medical School, 5214, Med Sci I, 1301 Catherine Road, Ann Arbor, MI 48109-0602, USA; e-mail: slkunkel@umich.edu

Nicholas W. Lukacs, Department of Pathology, University of Michigan Medical School, 5214, Med Sci I, 1301 Catherine Road, Ann Arbor, MI 48109-0602, USA

Anthony M. Manning, Signal Pharmaceuticals, Inc., 5555 Oberlin Drive, San Diego, CA 92121, USA; e-mail: amanning@signalpharm.com

Tracey J. Mitchell, Leukocyte Biology Section, Biomedical Science Division, Sir Alexander Fleming Building, Imperial College School of Medicine, London SW7 2AZ, UK; e-mail: t.mitchell@ic.ac.uk

Renate Nickel, Johns Hopkins University School of Medicine, Asthma and Allergy Center, 5501 Hopkins Bayview Circle, Baltimore, MD 21224, USA

Sem H. Phan, Department of Pathology, University of Michigan Medical School, 5214, Med Sci I, 1301 Catherine Road, Ann Arbor, MI 48109-0602, USA

Candy Robinson, DuPont Pharmaceuticals Company, Research and Development Experimental Station, P.O. Box 80400, Wilmington, DE 19880-0440, USA; has since moved to Cephalon Inc., Westchester, Pennsylvania, USA

Barrett J. Rollins, Department of Adult Oncology, Dana-Farber Cancer Institute, Harvard Medical School, 44 Binney Street, Boston, MA 02115, USA; e-mail: barrett_rollins@dfci.harvard.edu

Nancy H. Ruddle, Yale University School of Medicine, Department of Epidemiology and Public Health and Immunobiology, 815 LEPH, New Haven, CT 06520-8034, USA; e-mail: nancy.ruddle@yale.edu

Robert P. Schleimer, Johns Hopkins University School of Medicine, Asthma and Allergy Center, 5501 Hopkins Bayview Circle, Baltimore, MD 21224, USA

Syed Shahabuddin, Johns Hopkins University School of Medicine, Asthma and Allergy Center, 5501 Hopkins Bayview Circle, Baltimore, MD 21224, USA

Steven D. Shapiro, Division of Respiratory and Critical Care, Barnes-Jewish Hospital (North Campus), 216 South Kingshighway, St. Louis, MO 63110, USA; e-mail: sshapiro@imgate.wustl.edu

Cristiana Stellato, Johns Hopkins University School of Medicine, Asthma and Allergy Center, 5501 Hopkins Bayview Circle, Baltimore, MD 21224, USA

Susan C. Tseng, Department of Adult Oncology, Dana-Farber Cancer Institute, Harvard Medical School, 44 Binney Street, Boston, MA 02115, USA

Timothy J. Williams, Leukocyte Biology Section, Biomedical Science Division, Sir Alexander Fleming Building, Imperial College School of Medicine, London SW7 2AZ, UK; e-mail: tim.williams@ic.ac.uk

Preface

In November 1–5, 1998, the 9th International Conference of the Inflammation Research Association was held at The Hershey Lodge and the Convention Center at Hershey, Pennsylvania. In line with prior meetings this maintained the high academic standard and intimacy for detailed subjective discussions with colleagues. The program included morning symposia, afternoon posters and evening workshops. Of course there were many social moments and discussions with friends, new and old. All in all, it was a successful meeting and a heartfelt thanks are extended to the many participants and volunteers who gave so much of their time to the planning and staging of the conference.

The names of the supporters and helpers who contributed to the conference are listed. It is rather remarkable that a volunteer organization is able to undertake a conference such as this. As president of the Association, I extend my appreciation to everyone who contributed. I am very pleased that scientists from around the world were able to come and freely exchange their knowledge and views on the latest mechanisms and treatments of inflammatory disorders. As first began at the 8th International Conference, the last session on late breaking data/news on new drugs was of considerable interest. Also, the morning symposia and plenary lecture were all well received. I personally thank each of the speakers.

I also would like to thank the following companies for their generous donations and support: Chrysalis Preclinical Services Corp., Glaxo Wellcome Inc., Novartis Pharmaceuticals Corporation and Pfizer Inc., Central Research Division.

This book is a compilation of the talks delivered by the speakers of the morning symposia, summaries of the workshops, as well as the plenary lecture by Professor Timothy Williams.

L. Gordon Letts, President

The role of eotaxin and related CC-chemokines in asthma and allergy

Tracey J. Mitchell and Timothy J. Williams

Leukocyte Biology Section, Biomedical Science Division, Sir Alexander Fleming Building, Imperial College School of Medicine, London SW7 2AZ, UK

Introduction

The response to exposure to an aeroallergen in an allergic asthmatic consists of an initial bronchoconstriction associated with cross-linking of IgE on mast cells and the release of spasmogens, followed (except in mild reactions) by a late phase bronchoconstriction. The late phase bronchoconstriction is associated with an infiltration of airway tissue by inflammatory cells. These inflammatory changes are thought to underlie the airway hyper-responsiveness to spasmogens which is a characteristic of asthma.

Prominent amongst the inflammatory cells which accumulate in allergic reactions are eosinophils, which are thought to be major effector cells responsible for tissue injury and lung dysfunction by release of their highly cationic granular contents (EPO, ECP, MBP and EDN) and *de novo* secretory products such as peptidoleukotrienes. There is a direct correlation between lung dysfunction and the numbers of eosinophils in the lungs of asthmatic patients, and several animal models which demonstrate a link between eosinophils and lung dysfunction (although not invariably). Eosinophils are believed to have evolved as effector cells involved in local host defence to helminth parasite infections so that asthma and allergy can be regarded as aberrations of such defensive responses inappropriately triggered by otherwise innocuous agents. In this respect it is of interest that proteases secreted by helminth parasites to facilitate their access to, and survival in, host tissue can be potent allergens (e.g. digestive enzymes from house dust mites).

Allergic asthma is a major cause of morbidity and carries a significant risk of death from acute symptoms. Allergic asthma is a common disease, particularly amongst children, and the incidence is increasing worldwide for unknown reasons. One possibility suggested recently is that infant vaccination may skew the immune response towards an allergic profile. Asthma onset can also occur in adults, sometimes without the involvement of defined allergens. In these patients severe steroid resistant asthma is particularly difficult to manage.

Inflammatory Processes: Molecular Mechanisms and Therapeutic Opportunities, edited by L. Gordon Letts and Douglas W. Morgan
© 2000 Birkhäuser Verlag Basel/Switzerland

Eosinophil recruitment

Because of the potential importance of eosinophils in tissue damage and lung dysfunction there is considerable interest in mechanisms underlying their recruitment from the airway microvasculature. A key stage in this process is the local production of soluble chemical signals, "chemoattractants", which have an important role in stimulating the immobilisation and adherence of rolling eosinophils to microvascular endothelial cells, followed by transmigration into the tissue. This is achieved through signalling *via* chemoattractant receptors on eosinophils that mediate cytoskeletal changes within the cell and upregulation of adhesion molecules which engage complementary molecules on the endothelial cell surface (which may themselves be upregulated by cytokines generated in the tissue). A complex sequence of molecular interactions then takes place which results in migration of the cell through the endothelium and its basement membrane into airway tissue.

Eosinophil-selective chemokines

The observed eosinophil-rich infiltration occurring in allergic reactions implies the existence of endogenous eosinophil-selective chemoattractants, but until recently none of these had been identified. The complement fragments C5a and C3a, platelet activating factor and leukotriene B4 have chemoattractant activity for eosinophils, but they are also active on other cell types. A number of CC-chemokines have now been identified that act on eosinophils. The first CC-chemokine found to be chemotactic for eosinophils was RANTES. Thrombin-stimulated human platelets were found to release a protein with potent eosinophil chemotactic activity. Analysis of this protein identified it as RANTES, a CC-chemokine known also to stimulate other cell types such as monocytes and T cells [1].

In an attempt to identify putative endogenous eosinophil-selective chemoattractants, we assayed bronchoalveolar lavage (BAL) fluid from allergen-challenged sensitised guinea pigs using the accumulation of ^{111}In-eosinophils in the skin of naïve bioassay guinea pigs as an index. At 3–6 h post-challenge we could detect a factor in BAL fluid which induced eosinophil accumulation when injected intradermally. Edman microsequencing of the protein responsible revealed a novel 73 amino acid CC-chemokine, which we called "eotaxin" [2, 3]. Three distinct bands were seen on SDS-PAGE electrophoresis and we believe that these represent three glycosylation variants. The residue at position 70 could not be identified by protein sequencing but subsequent cloning of the gene showed that the encoded amino acid was a threonine, a potential O-glycosylation site. Recent unpublished observations in our group suggest that the attached sugars do have an important function in certain test systems. We found that eotaxin was highly active in stimulating eosinophil recruitment in guinea pigs and in stimulating guinea pig eosinophils *in vitro*. Interestingly the guinea pig protein also potently stimulated a calcium flux in human eosinophils [2] implying the existence of a human eotaxin and its receptor. Primers based on the guinea pig eotaxin sequence were used to clone a mouse eotaxin gene [4, 5], followed by human [6, 7] and rat [8, 9]. Functionally all the eotaxins are homologous in their role as highly selective and potent eosinophil chemoattractants. Despite their functional similarities, the eotaxin precursor sequences exhibit a high degree of cross-species sequence divergence for orthologous proteins. However, there is a 12 amino acid stretch at the C terminus that is conserved in eotaxin proteins from all species. Furthermore, the 3' untranstralated regions (3'UTRs) of the eotaxin genes cloned from different species all contain adenosine-uridine–rich elements (AREs). These AUUUA sequence motifs are present in the 3'UTR of many short-lived RNA species particularly those of cytokines and oncogenes [10, 11] and are known to confer mRNA instability. It is now recognised that the AREs represent an important regulatory mechanism for controling mRNA levels.

Recently two other CC-chemokines have been identified and due to their functional similarity to eotaxin they have been termed eotaxin-2 [12, 13] and eotaxin-3 [14, 15]. Like eotaxin, eotaxin-2 and eotaxin-3 appear to signal exclusively via the chemokine receptor, CCR3. However, structurally the three eotaxins are divergent. Eotaxin and eotaxin-2 exhibit only 39% identity at the amino acid level. Similarly, the identity at the amino acid level between eotaxin and eotaxin-3 is 36%. The eotaxin gene is located on chromosome 17q21.1-21.2 [16] in the CC-chemokine cluster, whereas eotaxin-2 and eotaxin-3 have been mapped to chromosome 7q11.2 [14, 17].

The monocyte chemoattractant proteins (MCPs) also belong to the CC-chemokine family and certain members of this sub-group have been identified as eosinophil chemoattractants, although unlike eotaxin, none act exclusively on eosinophils. Monocyte chemoattractant proteins -2, -3 and -4 function as eosinophil chemoattractants with varying potency. MCP-2 and -3 have similar efficacy [18] whereas MCP-4 is the most potent member of this family exhibiting an eosinophil chemotactic activity comparable to that of eotaxin [19–21].

Like eotaxin, the genes for the MCPs and RANTES have all been mapped to the CC-chemokine cluster on chromosome 17 [22]. This suggests that the CC-chemokine gene cluster arose recently in evolutionary terms, from a local gene duplication event. A recent study of the eosinophilic CC-chemokines (eotaxin, MCP-3, MCP-4 and RANTES) has compared the genomic organisation and transcriptional regulatory (promoter) regions of these genes [23]. Alignment of the four promoter regions reveals remarkable homologies around the TATA-box and the start-site of transcription. Several important transcription factor consensus binding domains that are known to be important in regulating inflammatory reactions are also present. Of note, nuclear factor kappa B (NF-κB) binding sites which are known to mediate the effects of TNFα and IL-1 [24]; γ-interferon response element (GRE) known (among others) to mediate IFNγ signalling; and glucocorticoid response elements

(GRE) which mediates glucocorticoid transcriptional regulation [25]. Glucocorticoid treatment has been shown to down-regulate expression of all four genes [16, 21, 26–29]. Although there are many similarities in the regulation of eotaxin, the MCPs and RANTES, clearly there are also important differences that lead to the observed differential effects on target cells and variation in tissue specific expression patterns.

Chemokine receptors on eosinophils

A G-protein coupled seven-transmembrane chemokine receptor, now designated CCR3, has been cloned from human [30–32], mouse [33, 34] and guinea pig [35] and found to be highly expressed on eosinophils. The three eotaxin proteins signal exclusively *via* this receptor. RANTES, with lower potency also signals *via* this receptor, but is non-selective. The monocyte chemoattractants MCP-2, 3 and 4 also stimulate this receptor, but are non-selective [36].

There is some controversy over the function of other chemokine receptors on eosinophils, particularly CCR1. Recently, it has been shown that a small subpopulation of individuals have eosinophils which respond highly to MIP-1α signalling through CCR1 [37]. All the individuals tested had eosinophils which responded highly to eotaxin, signalling through CCR3.

CCR3 has also been shown to be expressed on basophils [38] which are recruited to certain types of allergic reactions. Interestingly, a subpopulation of Th2 lymphocytes also express CCR3 [39–41] which is potentially important in maintaining the drive for allergic inflammatory reactions.

Chemokines in animal models of allergy

Eotaxin generation has been demonstrated in guinea pig [2, 42–45] and mouse [46] models of allergic inflammation. Studies in guinea pig showed eotaxin protein in lung tissue and BAL fluid 3 h after allergen challenge reaching a peak at 6 h [43]. Mice with targeted deletion of the eotaxin gene were shown to have a 70% reduction in lung eosinophils in sensitised mice 18 h after allergen challenge, but this effect diminished at later time points [47]. Another study using eotaxin knockout mice showed no detectable effect on eosinophil recruitment [48]. Clearly other ligands acting through CCR3 may be involved in the mouse. In addition, mouse eosinophils do have CCR1 so that MIP-1α may be involved. Animal species and strains, and the protocol used for sensitisation and challenge are all likely to be of importance in determining the precise role of specific chemokines and receptors. Recently it was shown that a single challenge of sensitised mice with cockroach antigen induced eosinophil recruitment and airway hyper-responsiveness which were unaffected by neutralising antibodies to MIP-1α or eotaxin. However, following allergen rechallenge airway hyper-responsiveness was suppressed by an antibody to eotaxin.

Constitutive eotaxin mRNA and protein were detected in naïve guinea pig lung, suggesting that eotaxin may maintain the basal eosinophil population of the lung in this species [3, 43]. More generally, eotaxin appears to be responsible for maintaining the population of eosinophils in the gut wall and this is depleted of eosinophils in the eotaxin knockout mice [47].

Chemokines in human asthma

Many chemokines have been detected in the airways of patients with asthma [49–52]. RANTES and eotaxin have been reported to be present in BAL fluid [53, 54] and recent studies have shown an increase in cells positively staining for eotaxin in airway wall biopsies [55–57]. Eotaxin staining is prominent in airway epithelial cells, microvascular endothelial cells and invading inflammatory cells [58]. Airway smooth muscle cells are also known to constitutively express CC-chemokines, including eotaxin [59, 60] and RANTES [61]. Ligands operating *via* CCR3 appear to have an important role in regulating eosinophil recruitment into the asthmatic lung, but this remains to be established clinically.

Interactions between chemokines and cytokines

There is considerable evidence that Th2 lymphocytes, originally described in the mouse [62] have a central role in regulating allergic inflammatory reactions [63]. The means whereby these cells control eosinophil recruitment has been under investigation for a considerable time. The observation that many cell types in the lung appear to be induced to express eotaxin highlights the important relationship between Th2 cells and other cell types. Thus, there have been several investigations of the potential of the Th2-cell-derived cytokines to switch on the eotaxin gene in other cell types. Adoptively transferred Th2 cells have been demonstrated to induce eotaxin expression along with lung eosinophilia in allergen-challenged mice [64–66]. Th2 supernatant alone administered intranasally to naïve mice has also been shown to induce expression of eotaxin and RANTES [67]. Studies examining the effects of individual Th2-derived cytokines, have identified a pivotal role for IL-13 as a potent inducer of eotaxin expression [67, 68]. Another Th-2 derived cytokine IL-4, induces eotaxin expression by human fibroblasts [69, 70]. Neutralisation of IL-5 in guinea pigs was shown to suppress allergen-induced eosinophil recruitment without affecting eotaxin production [43]. Thus, IL-5 has other routes to controlling eosinophil recruitment (see below). The observation that a subpopulation of Th2 lymphocytes express CCR3 [39, 41] provides the further possibility of a positive feedback loop which can perpetuate eotaxin production and eosinophil recruitment.

Proinflammatory cytokines derived from Th1 cells can also induce expression of eotaxin. Stimulation of human dermal fibroblasts [71] and lung epithelial cells [27] by IFNγ in the presence of IL-1 and TNFα upregulates the production of eotaxin. The TNFα and IL-1 induction of eotaxin expression is diminished in a dose-dependent manner by the glucocorticoid dexamethasone [27].

Eosinophil release from the bone marrow

IL-5 has an established role in eosinophil differentiation and proliferation in the bone marrow [72] and in increasing eosinophil survival once the cells have been recruited to an inflammatory site [73]. The role of IL-5 as a chemoattractant involved in local tissue eosinophil recruitment is more controversial and, at least in guinea pig models, we found IL-5 to be a poor chemoattractant *in vivo* compared to the potent effects of eotaxin [42]. IL-5 does however, induce acute release of eosinophils from the bone marrow [42, 74] and the resultant blood eosinophilia has a marked enhancing effect on the numbers of eosinophils recruited to tissues in response to eotaxin [42]. Interestingly, intravenously-injected eotaxin can also induce the release of the bone marrow eosinophil and shows marked synergism with IL-5 [75].

Conclusion

Research over recent years has resulted in an increasing insight into mechanisms involved in allergic inflammation. In particular, work on eotaxin and other CC-chemokines acting through CCR3 has provided a working hypothesis to explain mechanisms involved in eosinophil recruitment and the links between Th2 lymphocytes regulating allergic inflammation and eosinophils, believed to be major effector cells of tissue damage. Small molecule antagonists of CCR3 could provide an effective therapy for asthma and allergy in preventing eosinophil recruitment and the ensuing pathogenesis associated with their recruitment and activation in tissue.

Acknowledgements
T.J. Mitchell and T.J. Williams are supported by the National Asthma Campaign (NAC), UK. We are grateful to the NAC and the Wellcome Trust for generously supporting our research.

References

1   Kameyoshi Y, Dorschner A, Mallet AI, Christophers E, Schroder JM (1992) Cytokine RANTES released by thrombin-stimulated platelets is a potent attractant for human eosinophils. *J Exp Med* 176 (2): 587–592

2   Jose PJ, Griffiths-Johnson DA, Collins PD et al (1994) Eotaxin: a potent chemoattractant cytokine detected in a guinea-pig model of allergic airways inflammation. *J Exp Med* 179: 881–887

3   Jose PJ, Adcock IM, Griffiths-Johnson DA et al (1994) Eotaxin: cloning of an eosinophil chemoattractant cytokine and increased mRNA expression in allergen-challenged guinea-pig lungs. *Biochem Biophys Res Commun* 205 (1): 788–794

4   Rothenberg ME, Luster AD, Leder P (1995) Murine eotaxin: an eosinophil chemoattractant inducible in endothelial cells and in interleukin 4-induced tumour suppression. *Proc Natl Acad Sci USA* 92: 8960–8964

5   Gonzalo JA, Jia GQ, Aguirre V et al (1996) Mouse eotaxin expression parallels eosinophil accumulation during lung allergic inflammation but it is not restricted to a Th2-type response. *Immunity* 4 (1): 1–14

6   Ponath PD, Qin S, Ringler DJ et al (1996) Cloning of the human eosinophil chemoattractant, eotaxin. Expression, receptor binding, and functional properties suggest a mechanism for the selective recruitment of eosinophils. *J Clin Invest* 97: 604–612

7   Garcia-Zepeda EA, Rothenberg ME, Ownbey RT, Celestin J, Leder P, Luster AD (1996) Human eotaxin is a specific chemoattractant for eosinophil cells and provides a new mechanism to explain tissue eosinophilia. *Nat Med* 2 (4): 449–56

8   Williams CMM, Newton DJ, Wilson SA, Williams TJ, Coleman JW, Flanagan BF (1998) Conserved structure and tissue expression of rat eotaxin. *Immunogenetics* 47: 178–180

9   Ishi Y, Shirato M, Nomura A et al (1998) Cloning of rat eotaxin: ozone inhalation increases mRNA and protein expression in lungs of brown Norway rats. *Am J Physiol* 274 (1 Pt 1): L171–176

10   Shaw G, Kamen R (1986) A conserved AU sequence from the 3' untranslated region of GM-CSF mRNA mediates selective mRNA degradation. *Cell* 46 (5): 659–667

11   Chen CY, Shyu AB (1995) AU-rich elements: characterization and importance in mRNA degradation. *Trends Biochem Sci* 20 (11): 465–470

12   Forssmann U, Uguccioni M, Loetscher P et al (1997) Eotaxin-2, a novel CC chemokine that is selective for the chemokine receptor CCR3, and acts like eotaxin on human eosinophil and basophil leukocytes. *J Exp Med* 185 (12): 2171–2176

13   White JR, Imburgia C, Dul E et al (1997) Cloning and functional characterization of a novel human CC chemokine that binds to the CCR3 receptor and activates human eosinophils. *J Leukoc Biol* 62: 667–675

14   Kitaura M, Suzuki N, Imai T et al (1999) Molecular cloning of a novel human CC chemokine (Eotaxin-3) that is a functional ligand of CC chemokine receptor 3. *J Biol Chem* 274 (39): 27975–27980

15   Shinkai A, Yoshisue H, Koike M et al (1999) A novel human CC chemokine, eotaxin-

3, which is expressed in IL-4- stimulated vascular endothelial cells, exhibits potent activity toward eosinophils. *J Immunol* 163 (3): 1602–1610

16 Garcia-Zepeda EA, Rothenberg ME, Weremowicz S, Sarafi MN, Morton CC, Luster AD (1997) Genomic organization, complete sequence, and chromosomal location of the gene for human eotaxin (SCYA11) , an eosinophil-specific CC chemokine. *Genomics* 41 (3): 471–476

17 Nomiyama H, Osborne LR, Imai T et al (1998) Assignment of the human CC chemokine MPIF-2/eotaxin-2 (SCYA24) to chromosome 7q11.23. *Genomics* 49 (2): 339–340

18 Weber M, Uguccioni M, Ochensberger B, Baggiolini M, Clark-Lewis I, Dahinden CA (1995) Monocyte chemotactic protein MCP-2 activates human basophil and eosinophil leukocytes similar to MCP-3. *J Immunol* 154 (8): 4166–4172

19 Garcia-Zepeda EA, Combadiere C, Rothenberg ME et al (1996) Human monocyte chemoattractant protein (MCP)-4 is a novel CC chemokine with activities on monocytes, eosinophils, and basophils induced in allergic and nonallergic inflammation that signals through the CC chemokine receptors (CCR)-2 and -3. *J Immunol* 157 (12): 5613–5626

20 Uguccioni M, Loetscher P, Forssmann U et al (1996) Monocyte chemotactic protein 4 (MCP-4), a novel structural and functional analogue of MCP-3 and eotaxin. *J Exp Med* 183: 2379–2384

21 Stellato C, Collins P, Ponath PD et al (1997) Production of the novel C-C chemokine MCP-4 by airway cells and comparison of its biological activity to other C-C chemokines. *J Clin Invest* 99 (5): 926–936

22 Naruse K, Ueno M, Satoh T et al (1996) A YAC contig of the human CC chemokine genes clustered on chromosome 17q11.2. *Genomics* 34 (2): 236–240

23 Hein H, Schluter C, Kulke R, Christophers E, Schroder JM, Bartels J (1999) Genomic organization, sequence analysis and transcriptional regulation of the human MCP-4 chemokine gene (SCYA13) in dermal fibroblasts: a comparison to other eosinophilic beta-chemokines. *Biochem Biophys Res Commun* 255 (2): 470–476

24 Ueda A, Okuda K, Ohno S et al (1994) NF-kappa B and Sp1 regulate transcription of the human monocyte chemoattractant protein-1 gene. *J Immunol* 153 (5): 2052–2063

25 Beato M (1989) Gene regulation by steroid hormones. *Cell* 56 (3): 335–344

26 Hein H, Schluter C, Kulke R, Christophers E, Schroder JM, Bartels J (1997) Genomic organization, sequence, and transcriptional regulation of the human eotaxin gene. *Biochem Biophys Res Commun* 237 (3): 537–542

27 Lilly CM, Nakamura H, Kesselman H et al (1997) Expression of eotaxin by human lung epithelial cells: induction by cytokines and inhibition by glucocorticoids. *J Clin Invest* 99 (7): 1767–1773

28 Stellato C, Beck LA, Gorgone GA et al (1995) Expression of the chemokine RANTES by a human bronchial epithelial cell line. Modulation by cytokines and glucocorticoids. *J Immunol* 155 (1): 410–418

29 Kwon OJ, Jose PJ, Robbins RA, Schall TJ, Williams TJ, Barnes PJ (1995) Glucocorti-

coid inhibition of RANTES expression in human lung epithelial cells. *Am J Respir Cell Mol Biol* 12 (5): 488–496

30 Ponath PD, Qin S, Post TW et al (1996) Molecular cloning and characterization of a human eotaxin receptor expressed selectively on eosinophils. *J Exp Med* 183: 2437–2448

31 Daugherty BL, Siciliano SJ, DeMartino JA, Malkowitz L, Sirotina A, Springer MS (1996) Cloning, expression, and characterization of the human eosinophil eotaxin receptor. *J Exp Med* 183: 2349–2354

32 Kitaura M, Nakajima T, Imai T et al (1996) Molecular cloning of human eotaxin, an eosinophil-selective CC chemokine, and identification of a specific eosinophil eotaxin receptor, CC chemokine receptor 3. *J Biol Chem* 271 (13): 7725–7730

33 Gao J-L, Sen AI, Kitaura M et al (1996) Identification of a mouse eosinophil receptor for the CC chemokine eotaxin. *Biochem Biophys Res Commun* 223: 679–684

34 Post TW, Bozic CR, Rothenberg ME, Luster AD, Gerard N, Gerard C (1995) Molecular characterization of two murine eosinophil beta chemokine receptors. *J Immunol* 155 (11): 5299–5305

35 Sabroe I, Conroy DM, Gerard NP et al (1998) Cloning and characterization of the guinea pig eosinophil eotaxin receptor, CCR3: blockade using a monoclonal antibody *in vivo. J Immunol* 161: 6139–6147

36 Heath H, Qin S, Rao P et al (1997) Chemokine receptor usage by eosinophils. The importance of CCR3 demonstrated using an antagonistic monoclonal antibody. *J Clin Invest* 99: 178–184

37 Sabroe I, Hartnell A, Jopling LA et al (1999) Differential regulation of eosinophil chemokine signalling via CCR3 and non-CCR3 pathways. *J Immunol* 162: 2946–2955

38 Uguccioni M, Mackay CR, Ochensberger B et al (1997) High expression of the chemokine receptor CCR3 in human blood basophils. Role in activation by eotaxin, MCP-4, and other chemokines. *J Clin Invest* 100 (5): 1137–1143

39 Sallusto F, Mackay CR, Lanzavecchia A (1997) Selective expression of the eotaxin receptor CCR3 by human T helper 2 cells. *Science* 277 (5334): 2005–2007

40 Gerber BO, Zanni MP, Uguccioni M et al (1997) Functional expression of the eotaxin receptor CCR3 in T lymphocytes co-localizing with eosinophils. *Current Biology* 7: 836–843

41 Bonecchi R, Bianchi G, Bordignon PP et al (1998) Differential expression of chemokine receptors and chemotactic responsiveness of type 1 T helper cells (Th1s) and Th2s. *J Exp Med* 187 (1): 129–134

42 Collins PD, Marleau S, Griffiths-Johnson DA, Jose PJ, Williams TJ (1995) Cooperation between interleukin-5 and the chemokine eotaxin to induce eosinophil accumulation *in vivo. J Exp Med* 182: 1169–1174

43 Humbles AA, Conroy DM, Marleau S et al (1997) Kinetics of eotaxin generation and its relationship to eosinophil accumulation in allergic airways disease: analysis in a guinea pig model *in vivo. J Exp Med* 186 (4): 601–612

44 Griffiths-Johnson DA, Collins PD, Rossi AG, Jose PJ, Williams TJ (1993) The

chemokine, eotaxin, activates guinea-pig eosinophils *in vitro* and causes their accumulation into the lung *in vivo*. *Biochem Biophys Res Commun* 197 (3): 1167–1172

45 Rothenberg ME, Luster AD, Lilly CM, Drazen JM, Leder P (1995) Constitutive and allergen-induced expression of eotaxin mRNA in the guinea pig lung. *J Exp Med* 181 (3): 1211–1216

46 MacLean JA, Ownbey R, Luster AD (1996) T cell-dependent regulation of eotaxin in antigen-induced pulmonary eosinophila. *J Exp Med* 184 (4): 1461–1469

47 Rothenberg ME, MacLean JA, Pearlman E, Luster AD, Leder P (1997) Targeted disruption of the chemokine eotaxin partially reduces antigen-induced tissue eosinophilia. *J Exp Med* 185 (4): 1–6

48 Yang Y, Loy J, Ryseck RP, Carrasco D, Bravo R (1998) Antigen-induced eosinophilic lung inflammation develops in mice deficient in chemokine eotaxin. *Blood* 92 (10): 3912–3923

49 Sousa AR, Lane SJ, Nakhosteen JA, Yoshimura T, Lee TH, Poston RN (1994) Increased expression of the monocyte chemoattractant protein-1 in bronchial tissue from asthmatic subjects. *Am J Respir Cell Mol Biol* 10 (2): 142–147

50 Humbert M, Ying S, Corrigan C et al (1997) Bronchial mucosal expression of the genes encoding chemokines RANTES and MCP-3 in symptomatic atopic and nonatopic asthmatics: relationship to the eosinophil-active cytokines interleukin (IL)-5, granulocyte macrophage-colony-stimulating factor, and IL-3. *Am J Respir Cell Mol Biol* 16 (1): 1–8

51 Luster AD, Rothenberg ME (1997) Role of the monocyte chemoattractant protein and eotaxin subfamily of chemokines in allergic inflammation. *J Leukoc Biol* 62 (5): 620–633

52 Alam R, York J, Boyars M et al (1996) Increased MCP-1, RANTES, and MIP-1a in bronchoalveolar lavage fluid of allergic asthmatic patients. *Am J Crit Care Med* 153: 1398–1404

53 Lamkhioued B, Renzi PM, Abi-Younes S et al (1997) Increased expression of eotaxin in bronchoalveolar lavage and airways of asthmatics contributes to the chemotaxis of eosinophils to the site of inflammation. *J Immunol* 159 (9): 4593–4601

54 Berkman N, Krishnan VL, Gilbey T et al (1996) Expression of RANTES mRNA and protein in airways of patients with mild asthma. *Am J Respir Crit Care Med* 154 (6 Pt 1): 1804–1811

55 Brown JR, Kleimberg J, Marini M, Sun G, Bellini A, Mattoli S (1998) Kinetics of eotaxin expression and its relationship to eosinophil accumulation and activation in bronchial biopsies and bronchoalveolar lavage (BAL) of asthmatic patients after allergen inhalation. *Clin Exp Immunol* 114 (2): 137–146

56 Mattoli S, Stacey MA, Sun G, Bellini A, Marini M (1997) Eotaxin expression and eosinophilic inflammation in asthma. *Biochem Biophys Res Commun* 236 (2): 299–301

57 Taha RA, Minshall EM, Miotto D et al (1999) Eotaxin and monocyte chemotactic protein-4 mRNA expression in small airways of asthmatic and nonasthmatic individuals. *J Allergy Clin Immunol* 103 (3 Pt 1): 476–83

58 Ying S, Robinson DS, Meng Q et al (1997) Enhanced expression of eotaxin and CCR3 mRNA and protein in atopic asthma. Association with airway hyperresponsiveness and predominant co-localization of eotaxin mRNA to bronchial epithelial and endothelial cells. *Eur J Immunol* 27 (12): 3507–3516

59 Teruya-Feldstein J, Jaffe ES, Burd PR, Kingma DW, Setsuda JE, Tosato G (1999) Differential chemokine expression in tissues involved by Hodgkin's disease: direct correlation of eotaxin expression and tissue eosinophilia. *Blood* 93 (8): 2463–2470

60 Ghaffar O, Hamid Q, Renzi PM et al (1999) Constitutive and cytokine-stimulated expression of eotaxin by human airway smooth muscle cells. *Am J Respir Crit Care Med* 159 (6): 1933–1942

61 John M, Hirst SJ, Jose PJ et al (1997) Human airway smooth muscle cells express and release RANTES in response to T helper 1 cytokines: regulation by T helper 2 cytokines and corticosteroids. *J Immunol* 158 (4): 1841–1847

62 Mosmann TR, Cherwinski H, Bond MW, Giedlin MA, Coffman RL (1986) Two types of murine helper T cell clone. I. Definition according to profiles of lymphokine activities and secreted proteins. *J Immunol* 136 (7): 2348–2357

63 Robinson DS, Hamid Q, Ying S et al (1992) Predominant TH2-like bronchoalveolar T-lymphocyte population in atopic asthma. *N Engl J Med* 326 (5): 298–304

64 Li XM, Schofield BH, Wang QF, Kim KH, Huang SK (1998) Induction of pulmonary allergic responses by antigen-specific Th2 cells. *J Immunol* 160 (3): 1378–1384

65 Li L, Xia Y, Nguyen A, Feng L, Lo D (1998) Th2-induced eotaxin expression and eosinophilia coexist with Th1 responses at the effector stage of lung inflammation. *J Immunol* 161 (6): 3128–3135

66 Cohn L, Homer RJ, Marinov A, Rankin J, Bottomly K (1997) Induction of airway mucus production By T helper 2 (Th2) cells: a critical role for interleukin 4 in cell recruitment but not mucus production. *J Exp Med* 186 (10): 1737–1747

67 Li L, Xia Y, Nguyen A et al (1999) Effects of Th2 cytokines on chemokine expression in the lung: IL-13 potently induces eotaxin expression by airway epithelial cells. *J Immunol* 162 (5): 2477–2487

68 Zhu Z, Homer RJ, Wang Z et al (1999) Pulmonary expression of interleukin-13 causes inflammation, mucus hypersecretion, subepithelial fibrosis, physiologic abnormalities, and eotaxin production. *J Clin Invest* 103 (6): 779–788

69 Mochizuki M, Bartels J, Mallet AI, Christophers E, Schroder JM (1998) IL-4 induces eotaxin: a possible mechanism of selective eosinophil recruitment in helminth infection and atopy. *J Immunol* 160 (1): 60–68

70 Teran LM, Mochizuki M, Bartels J et al (1999) Th1- and Th2-type cytokines regulate the expression and production of eotaxin and RANTES by human lung fibroblasts. *Am J Respir Cell Mol Biol* 20 (4): 777–786

71 Bartels J, Schluter C, Richter E et al (1996) Human dermal fibroblasts express eotaxin: molecular cloning, mRNA expression, and identification of eotaxin sequence variants. *Biochem Biophys Res Commun* 225 (3): 1045–1051

72 Clutterbuck EJ, Hirst EM, Sanderson CJ (1989) Human interleukin-5 (IL-5) regulates

the production of eosinophils in human bone marrow cultures: comparison and inter-action with IL-1, IL-3, IL-6, and GMCSF. *Blood* 73 (6): 1504–1512

73   Yamaguchi Y, Suda T, Ohta S, Tominaga K, Miura Y, Kasahara T (1991) Analysis of the survival of mature human eosinophils: interleukin-5 prevents apoptosis in mature human eosinophils. *Blood* 78 (10): 2542–2547

74   Palframan RT, Collins PD, Severs NJ, Rothery S, Williams TJ, Rankin SM (1998) Mech-anisms of acute eosinophil mobilisation from the bone marrow stimulated by inter-leukin-5: the role of specific adhesion molecules and phosphatidylinositol 3-kinase. *J Exp Med* 188 (9): 1621–1632

75   Palframan RT, Collins PD, Williams TJ, Rankin SM (1998) Eotaxin induces a rapid release of eosinophils and their progenitors from the bone marrow. *Blood* 91 (7): 2240–2248

Signal transduction by the JNK group of MAP kinases

Roger J. Davis

Howard Hughes Medical Institute, Program in Molecular Medicine, Department of Biochemistry and Molecular Biology, University of Massachusetts Medical School, 373 Plantation Street, Worcester, MA 01605, USA

Introduction

MAP kinases are evolutionarily conserved proteins that are activated by a protein kinase cascade, including a MAP kinase kinase kinase, which phosphorylates a MAP kinase kinase, which in turn activates the MAP kinase by phosphorylation on Thr and Tyr residues. The primary sequence surrounding these phosphorylation sites serves to distinguish three major groups of mammalian MAP kinases. These include the Ras-activated ERK MAP kinases, which are characterized by the sequence TEY and the two stress-activated MAP kinases: p38 with the sequence TGY, and the c-Jun NH_2-terminal kinases (JNK) with the sequence TPY. This review will focus on the JNK group of MAP kinases.

The molecular cloning of JNK [1, 2] has led to the identification of a group of ten enzymes that are derived by the alternative splicing of three genes [3]. These JNK isoforms have different biochemical properties and they are differentially expressed in human tissues. JNK should therefore be thought of as a family of protein kinases [4]. The activaters of JNK have also been molecularly cloned. These are encoded by two genes, MKK4 and MKK7 [4]. Like the JNKs, these activators are also expressed as a group of alternatively spliced isoforms. This diversity of isoforms extends also to the upstream MAP kinase kinase kinases which activate MKK4 and MKK7. At present, at least 14 different genes have been identified to encode MAP kinase kinase kinases that may function within the JNK signaling pathway.

The JNK signaling pathway is arranged in a network together with the other MAP kinase pathways in mammalian cells (Fig. 1). These include the Ras-activated ERK MAP kinase pathway and the p38 and the JNK stress-activated MAP kinase pathways. In some cases, the activators are specific, in other cases there is promiscuity of signaling. Thus, by the selective use of different members of each pathway, the cell can respond to different stimuli by mounting selective or co-ordinated activation of MAP kinases to achieve an appropriate biological response.

Inflammatory Processes: Molecular Mechanisms and Therapeutic Opportunities, edited by L. Gordon Letts and Douglas W. Morgan
© 2000 Birkhäuser Verlag Basel/Switzerland

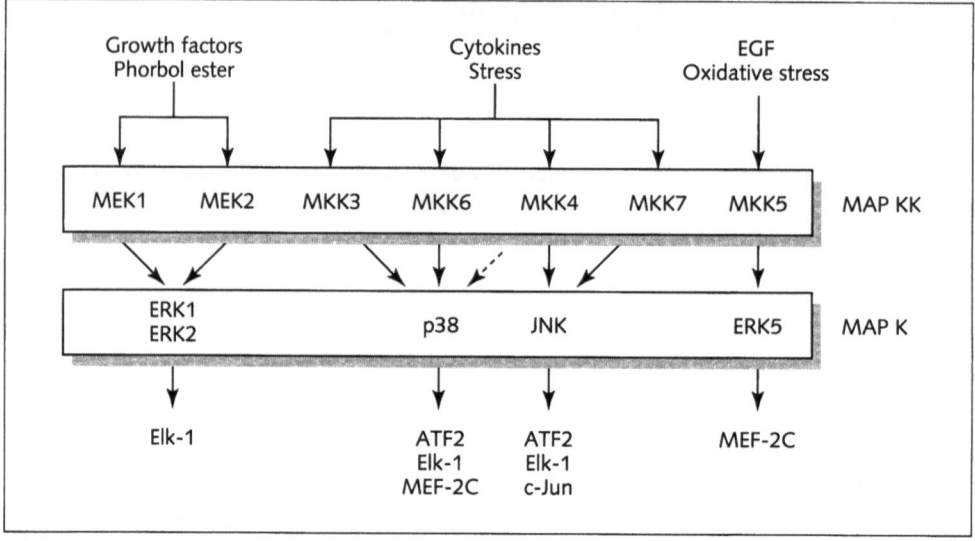

Figure 1

The mammalian MAP kinase signaling pathways are illustrated schematically. The ERK group of MAP kinases are activated by growth factors via a Ras-depedendent signaling pathway. The p38 and JNK signaling pathways are activated by many forms of environmental stress, including exposure to cytokines. The ERK5 pathway is activated by EGF and by oxidative stress.

Effect of the JNK signaling pathway on the activity of the AP-1 transcription factor

A major function of the JNK MAP kinases appears to be the regulation of AP-1 transcription activity. The mechanism of regulation is mediated, in part, by the phosphorylation of the activation domain of c-Jun, ATF2, and other proteins that can form dimeric AP-1 complexes. *In vitro* experiments indicate that the mechanism by which JNK regulates AP-1 transcription activity involves the binding of JNK to the activation domain of the AP-1 proteins c-Jun and ATF2. This binding interaction is necessary for substrate recognition by JNK and leads to the phosphorylation of two sites in the activation domain of c-Jun and ATF2. This phosphorylation causes increased transcriptional activity, presumably by inducing protein-protein interactions with co-activator molecules such as p300/CBP. As is the case for any model based upon *in vitro* experimentation, there is a significant question concerning whether this is an accurate description of the function of JNK *in vivo*.

Two lines of evidence support the contention that JNK is an activator of AP-1 transcription activity. First, this belief is consistent with both *in vitro* biochemical analysis and a large number of transfection experiments [4]. Second, in *Drosophila*, genetic studies demonstrate that a deficiency of JNK causes early embryonic death due to defects in morphogenesis [4]. Epistatic analysis demonstrates that an activated allele of Jun (created by replacement of the JNK phosphorylation sites with acidic amino acids) is able to rescue the morphogenic defect. This provides strong genetic evidence that c-Jun is a biologically relevant target of the JNK signaling pathway. However, these data do not directly address the role of JNK as a potential regulator of AP-1 transcription activity in mammalian cells. Recent studies of mice with disruptions of genes that encode components of the JNK signaling pathway have allowed a direct test of the hypothesis that JNK is a physiologically relevant activator of JNK signaling *in vivo*. The results of two studies are described below.

The first approach we used was to examine the phenotype caused by the knockout of one of the genes that encodes a JNK activator, MKK4 [5]. Southern blot analysis of genomic DNA demonstrated that we were able to obtain all of the expected genotypes (+/+, +/–, and –/–). The disruption we created is a null allele of MKK4, as demonstrated by Northern blotting and RT-PCR analysis of mRNA. Western blot analysis confirms that the MKK4 protein kinase is not expressed in homozygous cells, and a lower level of MKK4 expression was detected in heterozygous cells. In contrast, the substrate of MKK4 (JNK) is equally expressed in these cells. These MKK4-deficient cells provide an opportunity to test the role of the JNK signaling pathway in the regulation of AP-1 transcription activity *in vivo*. In these experiments, we compared the effect of two types of stimulus on both JNK activation and AP-1 reporter gene expression. These stimuli include an activator of the stress pathway (MEKK1) and an activator of the ERK MAP kinase pathway (Ras). Stress caused marked activation of JNK, while Ras is a modest JNK activator. This activation of JNK is eliminated in the knockout cells. Stress and Ras cause a similar induction of AP-1 transcription activity in wild-type cells. In contrast, there is a selective loss of stress-induced AP-1 transcription activation in the knockout cells. These data demonstrate that there is a stress-signaling pathway that requires JNK. However, JNK is not required for other signals, including Ras, that lead to AP-1 activation. Thus, JNK is required for some, but not all, signals that lead to AP-1 activation. Part of this complexity is accounted for by the fact that AP-1 is a group of dimeric transcription factors and that it is likely that different members of the AP-1 family mediate the effects of Ras and stress. In conclusion, the knockout of MKK4 (an activator of JNK) causes embryonic lethality and a selective defect in AP-1 transcriptional activity in response to stress.

A second example that illustrates the role of JNK in the regulation of AP-1 transcriptional activity is the knockout of the JNK3 gene, which is expressed in the brain [6]. This knockout is not lethal and mice with all the expected genotypes can be identified by Southern blot analysis. The disrupted gene is a null allele because the mRNA was not detected by Northern blotting or RT-PCR analysis. Furthermore, JNK3 protein kinase activity was not detected in the brains of the knockout mice. Importantly, we do not observe compensatory changes in the expression of other genes that encode JNK. We examined the effect of exposure to excitotoxic stress and we have particularly focused on the hippocampus and the expression and function of the AP-1 proteins c-Jun and c-Fos. Immunohistochemical analysis demonstrated that the expression of c-Fos and c-Jun in the hippocampus is extremely low. However, exposure to excitotoxic stress caused rapid induction of the AP-1 proteins c-Jun and c-Fos. No marked differences were detected between the wild-type and knockout mice. In contrast, immunohistochemical analysis of c-Jun phosphorylation demonstrated marked differences between the wild-type and knockout mice. Consistent with the low expression of c-Jun and low activity of JNK under normal conditions, we did not detect significant staining of the hippocampus. However, exposure to excitotoxic stress causes strong induction of phospho c-Jun in the dentate gyrus at early times and within the CA1 and CA3 regions of the hippocampus at later times. Importantly, no phospho c-Jun was detected in the hippocampus of the knockout animals. These data demonstrate that the knockout animals are defective in the stress-induced activation of JNK and phosphorylation of c-Jun in the hippocampus. To examine AP-1 transcription activity *in vivo*, we used a transgenic AP-1 reporter gene. These experiments demonstrated that the JNK3 knockout mice were defective in stress-induced AP-1 dependent reporter gene expression *in vivo*. These data demonstrate that JNK is not required in the brain for stress-induced expression of the AP-1 proteins c-Fos and c-Jun. However, JNK is required for c-Jun phosphorylation and AP-1 transcriptional activity. In this system, the transcriptional response leads to the induction of neuronal apoptosis, which is absent in the knockout mice. We conclude that the neuronal form of JNK (JNK3) is required for stress-induced AP-1 transcription activity and for stress-induced neuronal apoptosis.

Together, the evidence from studies of MKK4 and JNK3 knockout mice provides strong support for the hypothesis that JNK regulates AP-1 transcription activity *in vivo*.

Structural organization of the JNK signaling pathway

The structural organization of the JNK signaling pathway within the cell is not understood. For example, it is unclear whether all the components of the JNK cascade are separate within the cell and interact randomly through diffusion, or whether the cascade is assembled as a larger complex. Further studies are required to distinguish between these possibilities. However, recent progress in studies of the JNK signaling pathway has provided evidence that components of this signaling pathway may function within organized complexes [7]. The proteins that mediate

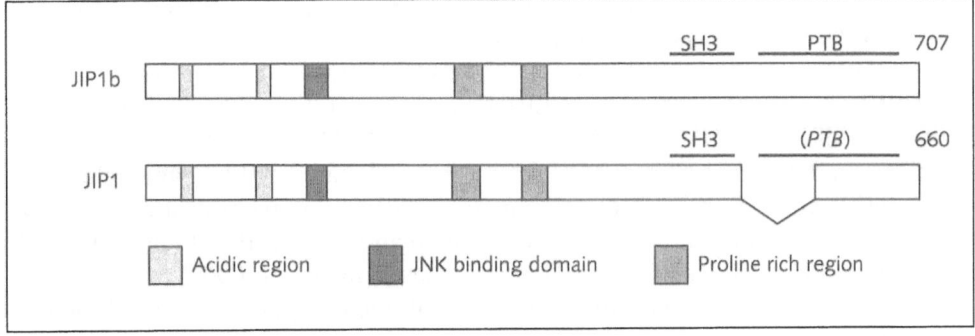

Figure 2
The JIP1 scaffold protein is expressed in two alternatively spliced forms. JIP1 differs from JIP1b by an in-frame deletion of sequences within the COOH terminal region. JIP1 has both an SH3 and a PTB domain in this COOH terminal region. The in-frame deletion disrupts the PTB domain in JIP1. The binding site for JNK is located within the NH_2-terminal region of JIP1 and JIP1b.

the structural coordination of such complexes are referred to as scaffold proteins [8].

We have examined whether scaffold proteins that bind individual components of the JNK signaling cascade are present in mammalian cells. Such proteins could serve to organize the JNK signaling pathway. These studies led to the molecular cloning of JIP1, a protein that binds stongly to JNK [9]. The JIP1 protein is expressed in two alternatively spliced forms that differ by the presence of an in-frame deletion in JIP1 that is absent in JIP1b. This in-frame deletion disrupts a PTB domain that is present in the COOH termional region of JIP1b (Fig. 2). To demonstrate that JIP1 can serve as a scaffold protein, it is necessary first to define what is meant by "scaffold" and second to show that JIP1 fulfills these criteria [10]. First, a scaffold protein should bind multiple components of the JNK signaling pathway. Second, the scaffold protein should enhance JNK activation by specific signals. Finally, the scaffold protein should inhibit JNK activation caused by other (irrelevant) signals.

The JIP1 protein does bind JNK. Co-immunoprecipitation analysis demonstrates that JNK1, JNK2, and JNK3 bind JIP1. However, the related protein kinases p38 and ERK do not bind JIP1 establishing that the binding of JNK to JIP1 is specific. To be a scaffold, it is necessary that JIP1 binds to additional components of the JNK cascade. We therefore examined the interaction of JIP1 with MAP kinase kinases. We found no co-immunoprecipitation of the activators of the ERK (MEK1 and MEK2) or p38 MAP kinases (MKK3 and MKK6) with JIP1. Similarly, we found no evidence for interaction of JIP1 with the JNK activator MKK4. However, binding of

MKK7 to JIP1 was observed. Reciprocal co-immunoprecipitation experiments confirm that JIP1 binds to MKK7, but not MKK4.

We also examined the binding of JIP1 to MAP kinase kinase kinases. No binding of JIP1 to c-Raf (an activator of ERK) was detected. Similarly, no binding was detected for the major class of JNK activators, MEKK. However, JIP1 was found to bind the mixed-lineage group of MAP kinase kinase kinases (MLK), which do function as activators of JNK. This interaction was confirmed in reciprocal co-immunoprecipitation experiments. Similar experiments demonstrated that binding to JIP1 was detected for a small sub-group of Ste20 kinases, including HPK1.

The JIP1 protein therefore interacts with multiple components of the JNK signaling pathway, including a Ste20-related protein kinase (e.g. HPK1), mixed-lineage kinases (e.g. MLK3), MKK7, and JNK. However, since these JNK pathway components can sequentially interact, it is unclear whether the binding to JIP1 is direct or indirect. To distinguish between these possibilities, we examined the binding of JNK pathway components in co-immunoprecipitation assays using JIP1 and a deletion mutant of JIP1 that fails to bind JNK. As expected, JIP1 but not the mutant JIP1 bound to JNK. However, MKK7, mixed-lineage kinases and the Ste20 protein kinase HPK1 bound to both the wild-type and the mutated JIP1 proteins. This analysis demonstrates that JNK binds to JIP1 independently of other components of the JNK cascade.

To further confirm that the binding of JNK pathway components occurs at independent sites on JIP1, we performed additional deletion analysis. These experiments demonstrated that JNK binds to the NH_2-terminal region, MKK7 to the central region, and the mixed-lineage kinases to the COOH terminal region of JIP1. These are direct interactions, since the binding is also observed using purified bacterially expressed proteins *in vitro*. We conclude from these experiments that JIP1 binds multiple components of the JNK cascade (Fig. 3). This fulfills the first criterion required for JIP1 to be a scaffold protein. However, there are two additional criteria that JIP1 must satisfy to qualify as a scaffold protein. JIP1 should suppress JNK signaling by irrelevant stimuli and it should enhance signaling by specific stimuli.

To test whether JIP1 can suppress JNK signaling, we examined JNK-dependent reporter gene expression and investigated the effect of JIP1 over-expression. These experiments demonstrated that c-Jun-dependent transcription was inhibited by JIP1 to an extent that was similar to that caused by mutation of the JNK phosphorylation sites located within the activation domain (Ser-63 and Ser-73). Similar observations were made using the transcription factor ATF2. A smaller inhibition was observed in experiments using Elk-1, probably because this transcription factor is also phosphorylated by other MAP kinases. In contrast to these observations, JIP1 did not inhibit many other transcription factors, including CREB, SP1, and VP16.

Probably the most important criterion for the function of JIP1 as a molecular scaffold for the JNK signaling pathway is that it should enhance the activation of

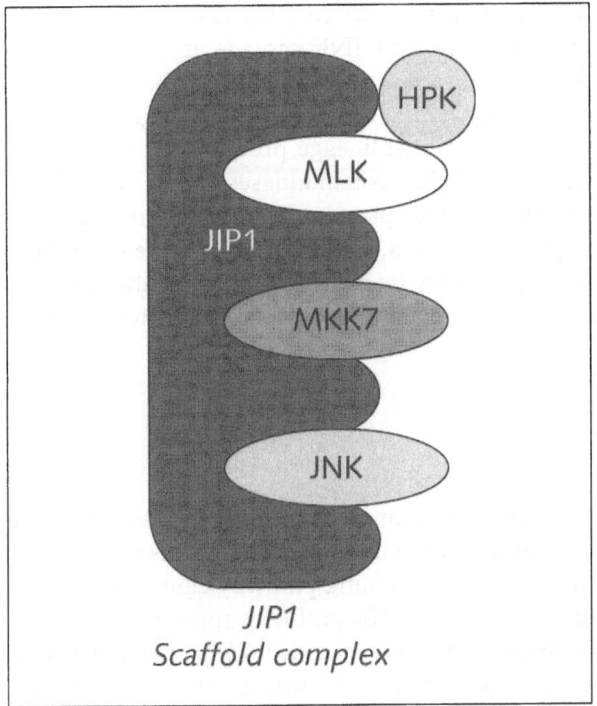

Figure 3

The JIP1 scaffold complex is illustrated schematically. JIP1 binds to Ste20-related protein kinase HPK1, the mixed-lineage group of MAP kinase kinase kinases, the MAP kinase kinase MKK7, and the JNK MAP kinases. JIP1 increases JNK activation mediated by the mixed-lineage kinase pathway and suppresses JNK signaling by other stimuli. This form of structural organization of signaling pathway components is likely to be important to achieve correct physiological regulation of JNK signaling.

JNK. JIP1 should act as a catalyst that increases signaling through the cascade in response to specific signals. To test whether JIP1 can increase JNK activation, we examined the effect of JIP1 expression on the activation of JNK by the mixed-lineage protein kinase MLK3. These experiments were performed using both wild-type JIP1 and the JIP1 mutant that does not bind JNK. Expression of these JIP1 proteins did not alter the low basal activity of JNK. MLK3 causes some increased JNK activity, which was strongly potentiated by JIP1, but not by the JIP1 mutant that fails to bind JNK. These data demonstrate that JIP1 can act as a positive regulator of JNK signaling mediated through the mixed-lineage group of MAP kinase kinase kinases.

The effect of JIP1 to enhance JNK activation is specific because the complexes formed by JIP1 involve only certain members of the JNK cascade at each step. For example, while both MKK4 and MKK7 can activate JNK, only MKK7 activity is potentiated by JIP1 and only MKK7 binds JIP1. Furthermore, although there are many MAP kinase kinase kinases, only the mixed-lineage protein kinases interact with JIP1. Similarly, only a limited group of Ste20 protein kinases interact with JIP1. These data indicate that JIP1 is a selective scaffold protein that is likely to be important for certain signals that lead to JNK activation. Other signals that lead to JNK activation do not employ JIP1. Such signals may be transmitted in the absence of a scaffold protein, or may be mediated by additional scaffolds that have not yet been defined.

Conclusions

The JNK signaling pathway represents an important mechanism that is used by cells to respond to envirnomental stress, including the inflammatory response. Gene disruption experiments demonstrate that the JNK signaling pathway causes activation of the AP-1 transcription factor. Activation of the JNK pathway appears to be coordinated by the interaction of components of the JNK cascade with scaffold proteins, including JIP1. The components of the JNK signaling pathway and the scaffold proteins represent potential targets for design of pharmacological agents that modify the inflammatory response in humans.

Acknowledgments
The work described performed in my laboratory was supported by grants from the National Cancer Institute and the Howard Hughes Medical Institute. I thank K. Gemme for excellent secretarial assistance.

References

1   Dérijard B, Hibi M, Wu I-H, Barrett T, Su B, Deng T, Karin M, Davis RJ (1994) JNK1: a protein kinase stimulated by UV light and Ha-Ras that binds and phosphorylates the c-Jun activation domain. *Cell* 76: 1025–1037

2   Kyriakis JM, Banerjee P, Nikolakaki E, Dai T, Rubie EA, Ahmad MF, Avruch J, Woodgett JR (1994) The stress-activated protein kinase subfamily of c-Jun kinases. *Nature* 369: 156–160

3   Gupta S, Barrett T, Whitmarsh AJ, Cavanagh J, Sluss HK, Derijard B, Davis RJ (1996) Selective interaction of JNK protein kinase isoforms with transcription factors. *EMBO J* 15: 2760–2770

4   Ip YT, Davis RJ (1998) Signal transduction by the c-Jun NH2-terminal kinase (JNK) – from inflammation to development. *Curr Opin Cell Biol* 10: 205–219

5   Yang D, Tournier C, Wysk M, Lu H-T, Xu J, Davis RJ, Flavell RA (1997) Targeted disruption of the MKK4 gene causes embryonic death, inhibition of c-Jun NH$_2$-terminal kinase activation and defects in AP-1 transcriptional activity. *Proc Natl Acad Sci USA* 94: 3004–3009

6   Yang DD, Kuan C-Y, Whitmarsh AJ, Rincon M, Zheng TS, Davis RJ, Rakic P, Flavell RA (1997) Absence of excitotoxicity-induced apoptosis in the hippocampus of mice lacking the JNK3 gene. *Nature* 389: 865–870

7   Whitmarsh AJ, Davis RJ (1998) Structural organization of MAP kinase signaling modules in yeast and mammals. *Trends Biochem Sci* 23: 481–485

8   Pawson T, Scott JD (1997) Signaling through scaffold, anchoring, and adaptor proteins. *Science* 278: 2075–2080

9   Dickens M, Rogers JS, Cavanagh J, Raitano A, Xia Z, Halpern JR, Greenberg ME, Sawyers CL, Davis RJ (1997) A cytoplasmic inhibitor of the JNK signal transduction pathway. *Science* 277: 693–696

10 Whitmarsh AJ, Cavanagh J, Tournier C, Yasuda J Davis RJ (1998) A mammalian scaffold complex that selectively mediates MAP kinase activation. *Science* 281: 1671–1674

Cellular signaling to NF-κB: Role in inflammation and therapeutic promise

Marie Chabot-Fletcher

Department of Immunology, SmithKline Beecham Pharmaceuticals, 709 Swedeland Rd., P.O. Box 1539, King of Prussia, PA 19406, USA

Introduction

Recent advances in our understanding of the mediators involved in acute and chronic inflammatory diseases have led to new strategies in the search for effective therapeutics. Traditional approaches include direct target intervention such as the use of specific antibodies, receptor antagonists, or enzyme inhibitors. Breakthroughs in the knowledge of regulatory mechanisms involved in the transcription and translation of inflammatory mediators has led to increased interest in therapeutic approaches directed at the level of gene transcription. Of the transcription factors targeted for pharmacological intervention, NF-κB has drawn much interest in light of its role as a coordinating regulator in the expression of a variety of rapid-response genes involved in inflammatory and immune reactions. The activation of NF-κB, its migration to the nucleus, and its binding to DNA provide numerous potential points of intervention, some of which are discussed below.

NF-κB belongs to a family of closely related dimeric transcription factor complexes composed of various combinations of the Rel/NF-κB family of polypeptides. The family consists of five individual gene products in mammals, RelA (p65), NF-κB1 (p50/p105), NF-κB2 (p49/p100), c-Rel, and RelB, all of which can form hetero- or homodimers. The proteins share a highly homologous 300 amino acid "Rel homology domain" which contains the DNA binding and dimerization domains (Fig. 1). At the extreme C-terminus of the Rel homology domain is a nuclear translocation sequence important in the transport of NF-κB from the cytoplasm to the nucleus. In addition, p65 and cRel possess potent transactivation domains at their C-terminal ends [1, 2].

First identified in B cells as a protein which bound to a decameric oligonucleotide present in the κ-light chain gene intronic enhancer [3], these complexes have since been demonstrated to be present in an inactive form in the cytoplasm of all cells studied [1]. The activity of NF-κB is regulated by its interaction with a member of the inhibitor IκB family of proteins. This interaction effectively blocks the nuclear localization sequence on the NF-κB proteins preventing migration of the dimer to

Inflammatory Processes: Molecular Mechanisms and Therapeutic Opportunities, edited by L. Gordon Letts and Douglas W. Morgan

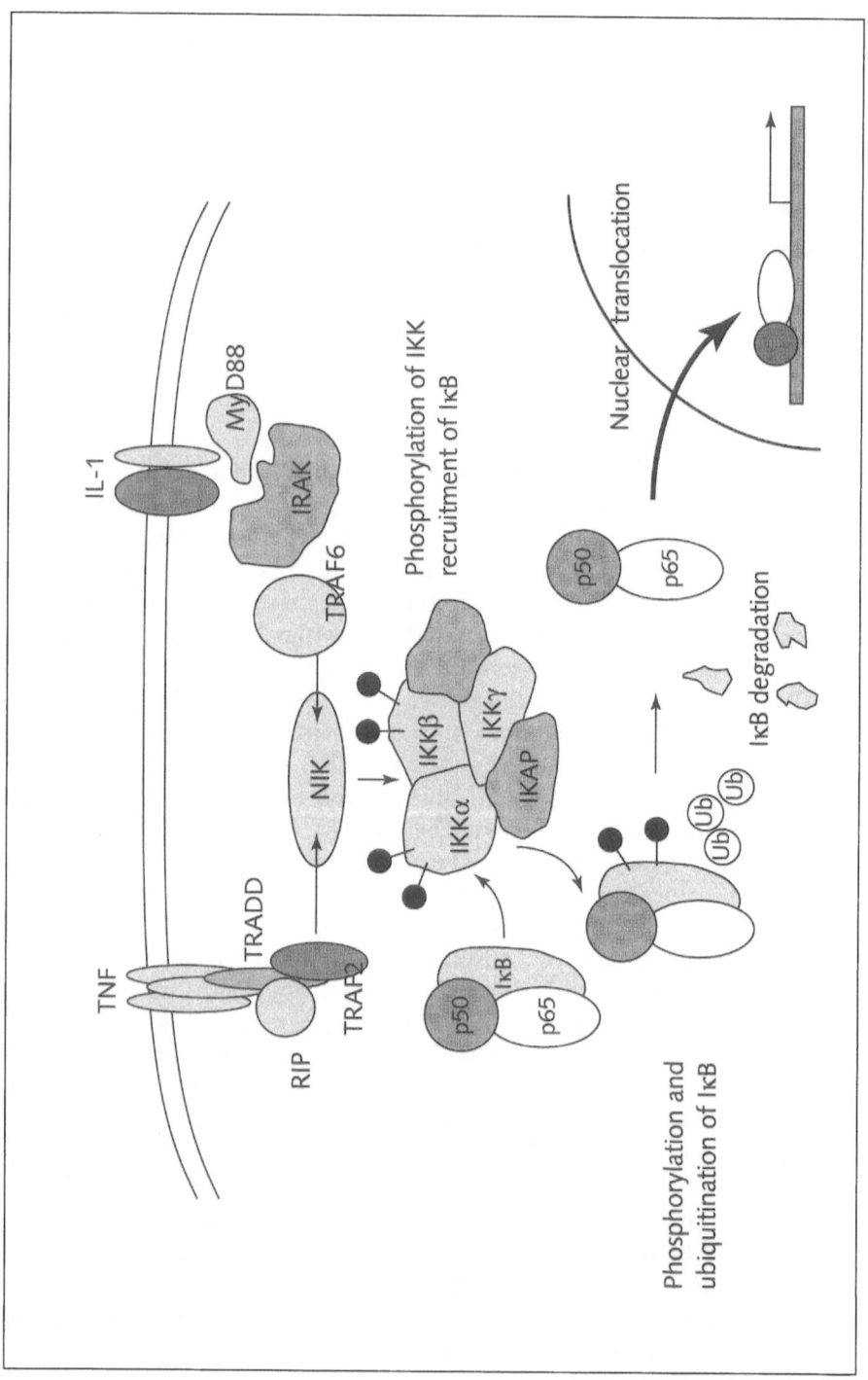

Figure 1
Pathways leading to the activation of NF-κB.

the nucleus [4, 5]. A wide variety of stimuli activate NF-κB, included are bacterial products (LPS), some viruses (HIV-1, HTLV-1), inflammatory cytokines (TNFα, IL-1), eicosanoids, T cell mitogens and physical stress [1, 2]. Common to all stimuli however, is the phosphorylation and subsequent degradation of IκB. Once free from IκB, the active NF-κB complexes are able to translocate to the nucleus where they bind in a selective manner to preferred gene-specific enhancer sequences. Included in the genes regulated by NF-κB are a number of cytokines, cell adhesion molecules, viruses, immunoreceptors, enzymes, and acute phase proteins [1, 2].

A role for NF-κB in inflammatory disorders

It is clear that NF-κB plays a key role in the regulated expression of a large number of pro-inflammatory mediators including cytokines such as IL-6 and IL-8 [6–8], cell adhesion molecules, such as ICAM and VCAM [9–11], and inducible nitric oxide synthase (iNOS) [12, 13]. Such mediators are known to play a role in the recruitment of leukocytes at sites of inflammation and in the case of iNOS, may lead to organ destruction in some inflammatory and autoimmune diseases [14, 15].

Asthma and airway inflammation

Evidence for an important role of NF-κB in inflammatory disorders is obtained in studies of asthmatic patients. Bronchial biopsies taken from mild atopic asthmatics show significant increases in the number of cells in the submucosa staining for activated NF-κB, total NF-κB, and NF-κB-regulated cytokines such as GM-CSF and TNFα compared to biopsies from normal non-atopic controls [16]. Furthermore, the percentage of vessels expressing NF-κB immunoreactivity is increased as is IL-8 immunoreactivity in the epithelium of the biopsy specimens [16].

NF-κB has also been shown to play a role in animal models of airway inflammation. Endotoxin-induced lung inflammation is associated with the activation of NF-κB in lung lavage cells after challenge [17]. Activation in the lung peaks 2 h after endotoxin injection and is temporally correlated with the expression of cytokine mRNA in lung tissue [18]. Furthermore, these responses are inhibited by pretreatment with N-acetylcystiene, an anti-oxidant inhibitor of NF-κB, in a concentration manner [18]. The activation of NF-κB in lung tissue is also seen in models of IgG immune complex-induced and ozone-induced lung inflammation [19, 20]. This activation may underlie the increased cytokine production and leukocyte infiltration characteristic of these disorders. In addition, inhaled steroids are known to reduce airway hyperresponsiveness and suppress the inflammatory response in asthmatic airways [21]. In light of the recent findings discussed below with regard to glucocorticoid action, one may speculate that these effects are mediated through an inhibition of NF-κB.

Inflammatory bowel disease

Recent studies suggest that NF-κB may also play a critical role in the pathogenesis of inflammatory bowel disease (IBD). Activated NF-κB is seen in colonic biopsy specimens from Crohn's disease and ulcerative colitis patients [22–24]. Activation is evident in the inflamed mucosa but not in uninflamed mucosa [22, 23] and is associated with increased IL-8 mRNA expression in the same sites [22]. Furthermore, corticosteroid treatment strongly inhibits intestinal NF-κB activation and reduces colonic inflammation [22, 24].

Animal models of gastrointestinal inflammation provide further support for NF-κB as a key regulator of colonic inflammation. Increased NF-κB activity is observed in the lamina propria macrophages in 2,4,6,-trinitrobenzene sulfonic acid (TNBS)-induced colitis in mice with p65 being a major component of the activated complexes [25, 26]. Local administration of p65 antisense abrogates the signs of established colitis in the treated animals with no signs of toxicity [25, 26]. As such, one would predict that small molecule inhibitors of NF-κB would be useful in the treatment of IBD. Consistent with this hypothesis, sulfasalazine, one of the most effective agents for treating IBD has recently been described as a potent and selective inhibitor of NF-κB [27].

Rheumatoid arthritis

Further evidence for a role of NF-κB in inflammatory disorders comes from studies of rheumatoid synovium. Although NF-κB is normally present as an inactive cytoplasmic complex, recent immunohistochemical studies have indicated that NF-κB is present in the nuclei, and hence active, in the cells comprising human rheumatoid synovium [28–30] and in animal models of the disease [31]. The staining is associated with type A synoviocytes and vascular endothelium [29]. Furthermore, constitutive activation of NF-κB is seen in cultured rheumatoid synoviocytes [32, 33] and in synovial cell cultures stimulated with IL-1β or TNFα [32, 34, 35]. Thus, the activation of NF-κB may underlie the increased cytokine production and leukocyte infiltration characteristic of inflamed synovium.

Glucocorticoid inhibition of NF-κB

The importance of NF-κB in immune and inflammatory disorders is also highlighted by recent studies showing that it may be a target for glucocorticoid-mediated immunosuppression and anti-inflammatory activities. Glucocorticoids have long been used as anti-inflammatory and immunosuppressive agents. However, the exact mechanisms whereby these drugs inhibit the transcriptional activation of pro-inflammatory cytokine and cell adhesion molecule genes was unclear in that glucocorticoid receptor binding sites were not found in the promoters of these genes. Common to many of these genes however, are NF-κB sites which have recently been shown to be involved in the glucocorticoid-meditated effects.

Glucocorticoids have been shown to inhibit the activity of NF-κB in response to stimuli through two separate mechanisms. First, a cross-coupling mechanism of inhibition exists between NF-κB and the glucocorticoid receptor such that this interaction prevents the binding of NF-κB to its target κB binding motifs [36–39]. More recently, glucocorticoids have been shown to inhibit the activity of NF-κB by inducing the expression of its natural inhibitor IκB-α [40, 41]. Thus, under conditions that normally cause the release of NF-κB, it quickly reassociates with newly synthesized IκB induced as a result of glucocorticoid treatment. As a consequence, the amount of NF-κB that translocates to the nucleus is reduced with a concomitant decrease in immune and inflammatory gene transcription. Clearly, this newly described mechanism of glucocorticoid action suggests that inhibition of NF-κB activation might be expected to exhibit the therapeutic benefits associated with glucocorticoid therapy.

Regulation of NF-κB function: points of intervention

The pathway leading to the activation of NF-κB presents many potential sites for intervention. Of these, the regulation of IκB function is a key target. Not only does this protein play a key role in the regulation of NF-κB but its function is in turn regulated by an activation cascade whose members may serve as pharmacological targets and are the focus of this review.

TNF and IL-1 signaling to NF-κB activation

In most cells NF-κB is held as an inactive complex in the cytoplasm through its interaction with a member of the inhibitor IκB family of proteins. The activation of NF-κB may thus be initiated through the binding of molecules such as TNFα and IL-1 to their respective receptors. Although TNF is able to bind two distinct receptors, the 55 kDa TNFR1 and the 75 kDa TNFR2 [42], gene knockout studies and receptor-specific agonist antibodies have demonstrated that TNFR1 is the major signaling receptor for TNF [43]. Upon TNF binding, receptor trimerization is induced resulting in the association with the TNFR1-associated death domain protein (TRADD) which subsequently recruits Fas-associated death domain (FADD/MORT1) protein and TNF receptor-associated factor 2 (TRAF2) [44, 45]. Whereas FADD is involved in signaling apoptosis, TRAF2 appears to be required for the activation of NF-κB and stress-activated protein kinases (SAPK) [44]. Therapeutic intervention by disrupting these protein-protein interactions would be expected to inhibit TNF-mediated activation of NF-κB.

In addition to its interaction with FADD and TRAF2, TRADD interacts strongly with the receptor-interacting protein (RIP), a serine-threonine kinase that is recruited to the receptor complex in a TNF-dependent manner [46]. Overexpression of RIP has been reported to induce both NF-κB activation and apoptosis [46] and RIP deficient cells are characterized by an inability to activate NF-κB in response to TNF stimulation [47]. Interestingly, a kinase inactive mutant does not block NF-κB activation [48] suggesting that inhibitors of RIP kinase activity would not block NF-κB activation in response to TNF stimulation. Thus, RIP and TRAF2 likely mediate the activation of NF-κB through their ability to interact either directly or indirectly with down-stream targets such as the NF-κB-inducing kinase (NIK).

With regard to IL-1, two cell-surface receptors for IL-1 have been identified and cloned. The biological effects of IL-1 are mediated through the type 1 receptor (IL-1RI) which is characterized by a single transmembrane domain, an extracellular immunoglobulin domain and a 212 amino acid cytoplasmic domain which is required for signaling. Upon the binding of IL-1 to the IL-1RI, the IL-1 receptor accessory protein (IL-1RAcP) is recruited to the complex. IL-1RAcP is required for IL-1 signal transduction, allowing IL-1-dependent activation of the IL-1 receptor associated kinase (IRAK) and SAPK [49–51].

IRAK was first identified as a novel serine-threonine kinase that could be co-immunoprecipitated with the IL-1RI after IL-1 treatment and required for IL-1 signaling [52–54]. Recruitment of IRAK to the IL-1RI/IL-1RAcP complex has recently been shown to be mediated by MyD88 [55, 56]. The kinetics of signaling complex formation suggest that MyD88 functions as an adaptor protein for the recruitment of IRAK. The interaction of MyD88 with the IL-1 receptor complex is thought to be mediated through a homophilic interaction through the conserved IL-1 receptor homology domain located at the C-terminal of MyD88 and in the cytoplasmic tail of the receptor [55, 57, 58]. In contrast, the N-terminal death domain of MyD88 mediates NF-κB activation upon overexpression and binds to IRAK suggesting a homophilic interaction mediated in part by the N-terminal death domains of both proteins [55].

MyD88 displays a high affinity for unphosphorylated IRAK and both proteins are recruited to the IL-1 receptor complex within 30 seconds of IL-1 treatment [55]. Association of MyD88/IRAK with the IL-1 receptor leads to the extensive phosphorylation of IRAK. This phosphorylation is likely to be mediated through autophosphorylation in that kinase negative mutants, although recruited to the receptor do not undergo phosphorylation [55]. MyD88 is unable to bind phosphorylated IRAK [55] and as such, upon phosphorylation IRAK disassociates from the IL-1 receptor complex and is able to interact with its down-stream target TRAF6.

A role for IRAK in IL-1-induced NF-κB activation is suggested from studies demonstrating that the overexpression of IRAK results in the activation of NF-κB

[55]. Furthermore, IRAK –/– fibroblasts have reduced NF-κB activation [59]. At this time it is not clear whether the kinase activity of IRAK is required for signaling. Studies reported by Yamin and Miller suggest that kinase activity may not be required, as is the case with RIP. These investigators have shown that the serine-threonine kinase inhibitor K-252b prevents IRAK phosphorylation but has no effect on its association with the IL-1R1 or on the subsequent degradation of IκB [60]. Thus, whether inhibition of IRAK is a viable mechanism through which to inhibit IL-1 mediated activation of NF-κB awaits further clarification of this signaling pathway using kinase inactive mutants and/or specific IRAK inhibitors.

NF-κB inducing kinase, a point of convergence

Downstream signaling in response to TNF and IL-1 stimulation is likely mediated through members of the TNF Receptor Associated Factor family of signal-transducing proteins, TRAF2 and TRAF6 in particular, and their subsequent interaction with downstream effectors. To that end, the NF-κB-inducing kinase (NIK) has been shown to be a TRAF2- and TRAF6-interacting protein [61]. NIK is an MAP3K-related kinase [62] that binds TRAF1, TRAF2, TRAF3, TRAF5 and TRAF6 [61]. Kinase-inactive mutants of NIK behave as dominant negative inhibitors that prevent TNF- and IL-1-induced activation of NF-κB [62, 63] and NIK overexpression induces the activation of NF-κB [62, 63]. As such, NIK is thought to play a critical role in the signal transduction cascade leading to the activation of NF-κB and is likely the point of convergence for the IL-1 and TNF signaling pathways to NF-κB activation.

The precise mechanism by which NIK is activated upon cell stimulation is not entirely clear. However, recent studies point to a mechanism involving the phosphorylation of a threonine residue within its activation loop. As is the case with many MAP3Ks, NIK is characterized by an activation loop located between subdomains VII and VIII in its kinase domains. Recent studies demonstrate that Thr-559 within this activation loop plays a critical role in regulating NIK activation [64]. Alanine substitution of Thr-559 inhibits NIK activity and when expressed, the mutant protein functions as a dominant negative inhibitor of TNF-induced NF-κB activation [64]. The kinase responsible for phosphorylation of Thr-559 within the NIK activation loop is not known although studies using the mutant NIK proteins suggest that auto- or trans-phosphorylation may be involved [64].

NIK's ability to activate down-stream signaling is thought to be mediated through the activation of the recently identified IκB kinases (IKK-α and IKK-β). The activation of the IKKs results in the subsequent phosphorylation of IκB and NF-κB activation. NIK has been reported to phosphorylate IKK-α preferentially over IKK-β [65–67] and phosphorylation has been mapped to Ser-176 within the IKK-α activation loop resulting in an increase in kinase activity [66]. A mutant form of IKK-α in which Ser-176 has been changed to alanine is not a substrate for NIK and acts as a dominant negative inhibitor of IL-1 and TNF-induced NF-κB activation [66]. The IKKs are also activated by MEKK1 although the mechanism underlying this activation is unclear [67, 68].

The IKK complex

It has been known for some time that upon cell stimulation, IκB-α is phosphorylated on Ser-32 and Ser-36 [69–72]. However, the kinase responsible for this activity was unknown. The studies of Chen and co-workers shed light on the identity of this kinase in studies which described a large multisubunit kinase (700 kDa) that phosphorylated IκB-α at Ser-32 and Ser-36 [73]. Subsequent studies demonstrated that the complex was also activated by MEKK1 although the kinases responsible for IκB phosphorylation remained anonymous [74]. The responsible enzymes were later identified to be IKK-α and IKK-β.

IKK-α and IKK-β were identified using both conventional protein purification efforts and in a yeast two-hybrid screen for NIK-interacting proteins [65, 75–78]. They were shown to be components of the large 700 kDa complex whose IκB phosphorylating activity was increased in response to cytokine stimulation. IKK-α is identical to a previously cloned serine-threonine kinase of unknown function known as CHUK [79, 80]. IKK-β was identified by virtue of its homology to IKK-α. The kinases are highly specific for the phosphorylation of serine residues and are known be activated by NIK and MEKK1 as discussed above [66–68].

Recently the NIK/IKK interaction was reported to be mediated through docking proteins present in the 700-kDa IKK complex. The IKK-complex associated protein (IKAP) was identified as a 150 kDa protein that can bind to NIK > IKK-α >> IKK-β and assemble them into an active kinase complex [81]. Similarly, IKK-γ was reported to interact preferentially with IKK-β and be required for IKK complex activity [82]. IKK-γ is the human homolog of the mouse NF-κB essential modulator (NEMO) identified by complementation cloning with an NF-κB unresponsive cell line [83]. As such these scaffold proteins play an important role in mediating signaling complex formation leading to the activation of the IKK. Once activated the IKKs are able to phosphorylate IκB resulting in the subsequent activation of NF-κB.

Although the phosphorylation of IκB is critical in the activation of NF-κB, this modification is insufficient to cause the dissociation of IκB from NF-κB [84–88]. Rather, inducible phosphorylation is thought to flag the protein for subsequent degradation *via* the ubiquitin-proteasome pathway [89–91]. Recent studies indicate that lysines 21 and 22 are critical in signal-induced, ubiquitin-mediated proteolysis [92, 93]. Mutation of these potential ubiquitination sites in IκB-α almost completely blocked the subsequent degradation of the protein and prevented the activation of NF-κB in response to stimulation. The critical role of ubiquitination in the regulation of downstream signaling suggests that inhibition of ubiquitin ligase may be a viable means of inhibiting the activation of NF-κB.

Once ubiquitinated the protein serves as a substrate for the 26S proteasome [90, 91]. This process is ATP-dependent and also has recently been shown to play a role in the processing of the NF-κB1 precursor (p105) to the p50 subunit [94]. Further evidence for a role of the proteasome in the degradation of IκB-α as well as its potential as a therapeutic target come from studies using the peptide Cbz-Ile-Glu(O-t-Bu)-Ala-leucinal (PSI), a specific inhibitor of the chymotrypsin-like activity of the proteasome. Micromolar amounts of this compound prevented activation of NF-κB [89], supporting that the activation of NF-κB is dependent on the constituitively active proteasome complex. Finally, one can envision inhibitors of NF-κB translocation to the nucleus as has been shown with nuclear localization peptides [95], or inhibitors of NF-κB/DNA binding.

Conclusion

NF-κB is a dimeric transcription factor which, upon activation undergoes translocation to the nucleus where it is involved in the regulated expression of a number of proinflammatory genes including cytokines and cell adhesion molecules. The recent finding that some of the anti-inflammatory properties of the glucocorticoids are mediated through an inhibition of NF-κB lends strong support to the proposal that an inhibitor of NF-κB will provide an anti-inflammatory therapeutic agent. Several potential pharmacological targets can be envisioned including inhibitors of the kinases involved in the regulation of IκB and hence NF-κB, inhibitors of IκB ubiquitination, and proteasome-directed inhibitors of IκB degradation. All in all, the complexity of the NF-κB activation process and of its interaction with DNA provide fertile ground for the development of a new generation of anti-inflammatory therapeutics targeted at the level of gene transcription.

References

1   Baeuerle P, Henkel T (1994) Function and activation of NF-κB in the immune system. *Ann Rev of Immunol* 12: 141–179
2   Kopp EB, Ghosh S (1995) NF-κB and Rel proteins in innate immunity. *Adv Immunol* 58: 1–27
3   Sen P, Baltimore D (1986) Multiple nuclear factors interact with the immunoglobulin enhancer sequences. *Cell* 46: 705–716
4   Baeuerle P, Baltimore D (1988) Activation of DNA-binding activity in an apparently cytoplasmic precursor of the NF-κB transcription factor. *Cell* 53: 211–217

5   Baeuerle P, Baltimore D (1988) IκB: a specific inhibitor of the NF-κB transcription factor. *Science* 242: 540–546

6   Mukaida N, MaheY, Matsushima K (1990) Cooperative interaction of nuclear factor-κB- and cis-regulatory enhancer binding protein-like factor binding elements in activating the interleukin-8 gene by pro-inflammatory cytokines. *J Biol Chem* 265: 21128–21133

7   Liberman TA, Baltimore D (1990) Activation of interleukin-6 gene expression through NF-κB transcription factor. *Mol Cell Biol* 10: 2327–2334

8   Matsusaka T, Fujikawa K, Nishio Y, Mukaida N, Matsushima K, Kishimoto T, Akira S (1993) Transcription factors NF-IL6 and NF-κB synergistically activate transcription of the inflammatory cytokines interleukin 6 and interleukin 8. *Proc Natl Acad Sci USA* 90: 10193–10197

9   Marui N, Offerman MK, Swerlick, R, Kunsch C, Rosen CA, Ahmad M, Alexander RW, Medford RM (1993) Vascular cell adhesion molecule-1 (VCAM-1) gene transcription and expression are regulated through an antioxidant-sensitive mechanism in human vascular endothelial cells. *J Clin Invest* 92: 1866–1874

10   Kawai M, Nishikomori R, Jung E-Y, Tai G, Yamanak C, Mayumi M, Heike T (1995) Pyrrolidine dithiocarbamate inhibits intercellular adhesion molecule-1 biosynthesis induced by cytokines in human fibroblasts. *J Immunol* 154: 2333–2341

11   Ledebur HC, Parks TP (1995) Transcriptional regulation of the intracellular adhesion molecule-1 gene by inflammatory cytokines in human endothelial cells. *J Biol Chem* 270: 933–943

12   Xie Q, Kashiwabara Y, Nathan C (1994) Role of transcription factor NF-κB/Rel in induction of nitric oxide synthase. *J Biol Chem* 269: 4705–4708

13   Adcock IM, Brown CR, Kwon O, Barnes PJ (1994) Oxidative stress induces NF-κB DNA binding and inducible NOS mRNA in human epithelial cells. *Biochem Biophys Res Commun* 199: 1518–1524

14   McCartney-Francis N, Allen JB, Mizel DE, Albina JE, Xie Q, Nathan CF, Wahl SM (1993) Suppression of arthritis by an inhibitor of nitric oxide synthase. *J Exp Med* 178: 749–754

15   Kleemann R, Rothe H, Kolb-Bachofen V, Xie Q, Nathan C, Martin S, Kolb H (1993) Transcription and translation of inducible nitric oxide synthase in the pancreas of prediabetic BB rats. *FEBS Lett* 328: 9–12

16   Wilson SJ, Wallin A, Sandstrom T, Howarth PH, Holgate ST (1998) The expression of NF-kappa-B and associated adhesion molecules in mild asthmatics and normal controls. *J Allergy Clin Immunol* 101: 616

17   Blackwell TS, Holden EP, Blackwell TR, DeLarco JE, Christman JW (1994). Cytokine-induced neutrophil chemoattractant mediates neutrophillic alveolitis in rats: association with nuclear factor κB activation. *Amer J Resp Cell Mol Biol* 11: 464–472

18   Blackwell TS, Blackwell TR, Holden EP, Christman BW, Christman JW (1996) *In vivo* antioxidant treatment suppresses nuclear factor-κB activation and neutrophilic lung inflammation. *J Immunol* 157: 1630–1637

19 Haddad E-B, Salmon M, Koto H, Barnes PJ, Adcock I, Chung KF (1996) Ozone induction of cytokine-induced neutrophil chemoattractant (CINC) and nuclear factor-κB in rat lung: inhibition by corticosteroids. *FEBS Lett* 379: 265–268

20 Lentsch AB, Czermak BJ, Bless NM, Ward PA (1998) NF-κB activation during IgG immune complex-induced lung injury; requirements for TNF-α and IL-1β but not complement. *Am J Pathol* 152: 1327–1336

21 Barnes PJ (1989) A new approach to the treatment of asthma. *New Eng J Med* 321: 1517–1527

22 Ardite E, Panes J, Miranda M, Salas A, Elizalde JI, Sans M, Arce Y, Bordas JM, Fernandez-Checa JC, Pique JM (1998) Effects of steroid treatment on activation of nuclear factor κB in patients with inflammatory bowel disease. *Br J Pharmacol* 124: 431–433

23 Rogler G, Brand K, Vogl D, Page S, Hofmeister R, Andus T, Knuechel R, Baeuerle PA, Scholmerich J, Gross V (1998) Nuclear factor κB is activated in macrophage and epithelial cells of inflamed intestinal mucosa. *Gastroenterol* 115: 357–369

24 Schreiber S, Nikolaus S, Hampe J (1998) Activation of nuclear factor κB in inflammatory bowel disease. *Gut* 42: 477–484

25 Neurath MF, Pettersson S, Meyer zum Buschenfelde K-H, Strober W (1996) Local administration of antisense phosphorothioate oligonucleotides to the p65 subunit of NF-κB abrogates established experimental colitis in mice. *Nature Med* 2: 998–1004

26 Neurath MF, Pettersson S (1997) Predominant role of NF-κB p65 in the pathogenesis of chronic intestinal inflammation. *Immunobiol* 198: 91–98

27 Wahl C, Liptay S, Adler G, Schmid RM (1998) Sulfasalazine: a potent and specific inhibitor of nuclear factor kappa B. *J Clin Invest* 101: 1163–1174

28 Handel ML, McMorrow LB, Gravallese EM (1995) Nuclear factor-κB in rheumatoid synovium; localization of p50 and p65. *Arthritis Rheum* 38: 1762–1770

29 Marok R, Winyard PG, Coumbe A, Kus ML, Gaffney K, Blades S, Mapp PI, Morris CJ, Blake DR, Kaltschmidt C, Baeuerle PA (1996) Activation of the transcription factor nuclear factor-κB in human inflamed synovial tissue. *Arthritis Rheum* 39: 583–591

30 Sioud M, Mellbye O, Forre O (1998) Analysis of the NF-κB p65 subunit, Fas antigen, Fas ligand and Bcl-2-related proteins in the synovium of RA and polyarticular JRA. *Clin Exp Rheumatol* 16: 125–134

31 Tsao PW, Suzuki T, Totsuka R, Murata T, Takagi T, Ohmachi Y, Fujimura H, Takata I (1997) The effect of dexamethasone on the expression of activated NF-κB in adjuvant arthritis. *Clin Immunol Immunopathol* 83: 173–178

32 Roshak AK, Jackson JR, McGough K, Chabot-Fletcher M, Mochan E, Marshall L (1996) Manipulation of distinct NFκB proteins alters interleukin-1β-induced human rheumatoid synovial fibroblast prostaglandin E2 formation. *J Biol Chem* 271: 31496–31501

33 Miyazawa K, Mori A, Yamamoto K, Okudaira H (1998) Constitutive transcription of the human interleukin-6 gene by rheumatoid synoviocytes; spontaneous activation of NF-κB and CBF1. *Am J Pathol* 152: 793–803

34 Fujisawa K, Aono H, Hasunuma T, Yamamoto K, Mita S, Nishiola K (1996) Activation

of transcription factor NF-κB in human synovial cells in response to tumor necrosis factor α. *Arthritis Rheum* 39: 197–203

35 Roshak AK, Jackson JR, Chabot-Fletcher M, Marshall L (1997) Inhibition of NF-κB-mediated interleukin-1β-stimulated prostaglandin E2 formation by the marine natural product hymenialdisine. *J Pharmacol Exp Therapeut* 283: 955–961

36 Ray A, Prefontaine KE (1994) Physical association and functional antagonism between the p65 subunit of transcription factor NF-κB and the glucocorticoid receptor. *Proc Natl Acad Sci USA* 91: 752–756

37 Mukaida N, Morita M, IshikawaY, Rice N, Okamoto S, Kasahara T, Matsushima K (1994) Novel mechanism of glucocorticoid-mediated gene repression. *J Biol Chem* 269: 13289–13295

38 Caldenhoven E, Liden J, Wissink S, Van de Stolpe A, Raaijmakers J, Koenderman L, Okret S, Gustafsson J-A, Van der Saag PT (1995) Negative cross-talk between RelA and the glucocorticoid receptor: a possible mechanism for the antiinflammatory action of glucocorticoids. *Mol Endocrinol* 9: 401–412

39 Scheinman RI, Gualberto A, Jewell CM, Cidlowski JA, Baldwin AS Jr (1995) Characterization of mechanisms involved in transrepression of NF-κB by activated glucocorticoid receptors. *Mol Cell Biol* 15: 943–953

40 Scheinman RI, Cogswell PC, Lofquist AK, Baldwin AS (1995) Role of transcriptional activation of IκBα in mediation of immunosuppression by glucocorticoids. *Science* 270: 283–286

41 Auphan N, DiDonato JA, Rosette C, Helmberg A, Karin M (1995) Immunosuppression by glucocorticoids: inhibition of NF-κB activity through induction of IκB synthesis. *Science* 270: 286–290

42 Tartaglia LA, Goeddel DV (1992) Two TNF receptors. *Immunol Today* 13: 151–153

43 Vandenabeele P, Declercq W, Beyaert R, Tiers W (1995) *Trends Cell Biol* 5: 392–399

44 Hsu H, Shu H-B, Pan M-P Goeddel DV (1996) TRADD-TRAF2 and TRADD-FADD interactions define two distinct TNF receptor-1 signal transduction pathways. *Cell* 84: 299–308

45 Chinnaiyan AM, Tepper CG, Seldin MF, O'Rourke K, Kischkel FC, Hellbardt S, Krammer PH, Peter ME, Dixit VM (1996) FADD/MORT is a common mediator of CD95 (Fas/APO-1)- and TNF-receptor-induced apoptosis. *J Biol Chem* 271: 4961–4965

46 Hsu H, Huang J, Shu H-B, Baichwal V, Goeddel DV (1996) TNF-dependent recruitment of the protein kinase RIP to the TNF receptor-1 signaling complex. *Immunity* 4: 387–396

47 Kelliher M, Grimm S, Ishida Y, Kuo F, Stanger BZ, Leder P (1998) The death domain kinase RIP mediates the TNF-induced NF-κB signal. *Immunity* 8: 297–303

48 Ting AT, Pimentel-Muinos FX, Seed B (1996) RIP mediates tumor necrosis factor receptor 1 activation of NF-κB but not Fas/APO-1 initiated apoptosis. *EMBO J* 15: 6189–6196

49 Wesche H, Korherr C, Kracht M, Falk W, Resch K, Martin MU (1997) The interleukin-1 receptor accessory protein (IL-1RAcP) is essential for IL-1-induced activation of inter-

leukin-1 receptor-associated kinase (IRAK) and stress-activated protein kinases (SAP kinases). *J Biol Chem* 272: 7727–7731

50   Huang J, Gao X, Li S, Cao Z (1997) Recruitment of IRAK to the interleukin 1 receptor complex requires interleukin 1 receptor accessory protein. *Proc Natl Acad Sci USA* 94: 12829–12832

51   Volpe F, Clatworthy J, Kaptein A, Maschera, B, Griffin A-M, Ray K (1997) The IL-1 receptor accessory protein is responsible for the recruitment of the interleukin-1 receptor associated kinase to the IL1/IL1 receptor I complex. *FEBS Lett* 419: 41–44

52   Martin M, Fleur Bol G, Eriksson A, Resch K, Brigelius-Flohe R (1994) Interleukin-1-induced activation of a protein kinase co-precipitating with the type I interleukin-1 receptor in T cells. *Eur J Immunol* 24: 1566–1571

53   Coston GE, Cao Z, Goeddel DV (1995) NF-κB activation by interleukin-1 (IL-1) requires an IL-1 receptor-associated protein kinase activity. *J Biol Chem* 270 16514–16517

54   Cao Z, Henzel WJ, Gao X (1996) IRAK: A kinase associated with the interleukin-1 receptor. *Science* 271: 1128–1131

55   Wesche H, Henzel WJ, Shillinglaw W, Li S, Cao Z (1997) MyD88: An adapter that recruits IRAK to the IL-1 receptor complex. *Immunity* 7: 837–847

56   Burns K, Martinon F, Esslinger C, Pahl H, Schneider P, Bodmer JL, Di Marco F, French L, Tschopp J (1998) MyD88, an adapter protein involved in interleukin-1 signaling. *J Biol Chem* 273: 12203–12209

57   Hultmark D (1994) Macrophage differentiation marker MyD88 is a member of the Toll/IL-1 receptor family. *Biochem Biophys Res Commun* 199: 144–146

58   Hardiman G, Rock FL, Balasubramanian S, Kastelein RA, Bazan JF (1996) Molecular characterization and modular analysis of human MyD88. *Oncogene* 13: 2467–2475

59   Kanakaraj P, Schafer PH, Cavender DE, Wu Y, Ngo K, Grealish PF, Wadsworth SA, Peterson PA, Siekierka JJ, Harris CA, Fung-Leung W-P (1998) Interleukin (IL)-1 receptor-associated kinase (IRAK) requirement for optimal induction of multiple IL-1 signaling pathways and IL-6 production. *J Exp Med* 187: 2073–2079

60   Yamin TT, Miller DK (1997) The interleukin-1 receptor-associated kinase is degraded by proteasomes following its phosphorylation. *J Biol Chem* 272: 21540–21547

61   Song HY, Regnier CH, Kirschning CJ, Goeddel DV, Rothe M (1997) Tumor necrosis factor (TNF)-mediated kinase cascades: Bifurcation of nuclear factor-κB and c-jun N-terminal kinase (JNK/SAPK) pathways at the TNF receptor-associated factor 2. *Proc Natl Acad Sci USA* 94: 9792–9796

62   Malinin NL, Boldin MP, Kovalenko AV, Wallach D (1997) MAP3K-related kinase involved in NF-κB induction by TNF, CD95 and IL-1. *Nature* 385: 540–544

63   Natoli G, Costanzo A, Moretti F, Fulco M, Balsano C, Levero M (1997) Tumor necrosis factor (TNF) receptor 1 signaling downstream of TNF receptor-associated factor 2. *J Biol Chem* 272: 26079–26082

64   Lin X, Mu Y, Cunningham ET, Marcu, KB, Geleziunas R, Greene WC (1998) Molecular determinants of NF-κB-inducing kinase action. *Mol Cell Biol* 18: 5899–5907

65 Regnier CH, Song HY, Gao X, Goeddel DV, Cao Z, Rothe M (1997) Identification and characterization of an IκB kinase. *Cell* 90: 373–383

66 Ling L, Cao Z, Goeddel DV (1998) NF-κB-inducing kinase activates IKK-α by phosphorylation of Ser-176. *Proc Natl Acad Sci USA* 95: 3792–3797

67 Nakano H, Shindo M, Sakon S, Nishinaka S, Mihara M, Yagita H, Okumura K (1998) Differential regulation of IκB kinase a and b by two upstream kinases, NF-κB-inducing kinase and mitogen-activated protein kinase/ERK kinase kinase-1. *Proc Natl Acad Sci USA* 95: 3537–3542

68 Lee FS, Peters RT, Dang LC, Maniatis T (1998) MEKK1 activates both IκB kinase α and β. *Proc Natl Acad Sci USA* 95: 9319–9324

69 Brown K, Gerstberger S, Carlson L, Franzoso G, Siebenlist U (1995) Control of IκB-α proteolysis by site-specific signal-induced phosphorylation. *Science* 267: 1485–1488

70 Brockman JA, Scherer DC, McKinsey TA, Hall SM, Qi X, Lee WY, Ballard DW (1995) Coupling of a signal response domain in IκBα to multiple pathways for NF-κB activation. *Mol Cell Biol* 15: 2809–2818

72 Whiteside ST, Ernst MK, LeBail O, Laurent-Winter C, Rice N, Israel A (1995) N- and C-terminal sequences control degradation of MAD3/IκBα in response to inducers of NF-κB activity. *Mol Cell Biol* 15: 5339–5345

73 Chen ZJ, Parent L, Maniatis T (1996) Site-specific phosphorylation of IκBα by a novel ubiquitination-dependent protein kinase activity. *Cell* 84: 853–862

74 Lee FS, Hagler J, Chen ZJ, Maniatis T (1997) Activation of the IκBα kinase complex by MEKK1, a kinase of the JNK pathway. *Cell* 88: 213–222

75 DiDonato JA, Hayakawa M, Rothwarf DM, Zandi E, Karin M (1997) A cytokine-responsive IκB kinase that activates the transcription factor NF-κB. *Nature* 388: 548–554

76 Zandi E, Rothwarf DM, Delhase M, Hayakawa M, Karin M (1997) The IκB kinase complex (IKK) contains two kinase subunits, IKKα and IKKβ, necessary for IκB phosphorylation and NF-κB activation. *Cell* 91: 243–252

77 Mercurio F, Zhu H, Murray BW, Shevchenko A, Bennett BL, Li J, Young DB, Barbosa M, Mann M, Manning A, Rao A (1997) IKK-1 and IKK-2: Cytokine-activated IκB kinases essential for NF-κB activation. *Science* 278: 860–866

78 Woronicz JD, Gao X, Cao Z, Rothe M, Goeddel DV (1997) IκB kinase-β: NF-κB activation and complex formation with IκB kinase-α and NIK. *Science* 278: 866–869

79 Connelly MA, Marcu KB (1995) CHUK, a new member of the helix-loop-helix and leucine zipper families of interacting proteins, contains a serine-threonine kinase catalytic domain. *Cell Mol Biol Res* 41: 537–549

80 Mock BA, Connelly MA, McBride OW, Kozak CA, Marcu KB (1995) CHUK, a conserved helix-loop-helix ubiquitous kinase, maps to human chromosome 10 and mouse chromosome 19. *Genomics* 27: 348–351

81 Cohen L, Henzel WJ, Baeuerle PA (1998) IKAP is a scaffold protein of the IκB kinase complex. *Nature* 395: 292–296

82   Rothwarf DM, Zandi E, Natoli G, Karin M (1998) IKK-γ is an essential regulatory sub-unit of the IκB kinase complex. *Nature* 395: 297–300

83   Yamaoka S, Courtois G, Bessia C, Whiteside ST, Weil R, Agou F, Kirk HE, Kay RJ, Israel A (1998) Complementation cloning of NEMO, a component of the IκB kinase complex essential for NF-κB activation. *Cell* 93: 1231–1240

84   Henkel T, Machleidt T, Alklay I, Kronke M, Ben-Neriah Y, Baeuerle PA (1993) Rapid proteolysis of IκB-α is required for activation of the nuclear transcription factor NF-κB. *Nature* 365: 182–185

85   Finco TS, Beg AA, Baldwin SA Jr (1994) Inducible phosphorylation of IκBα is not suf-ficient for its dissociation from NF-κB and is inhibited by protease inhibitors. *Proc Natl Acad Sci USA* 91: 11884–11888

86   Lin Y-C, Brown K, Siebenlist U (1995) Activation of NF-κB requires proteolysis of the inhibitor IκB-α: signal-induced phosphorylation of IκB-α alone does not release active NF-κB. *Proc Natl Acad Sci USA* 92: 552–556

87   Alkalay I, Yaron A, Hatsubai A, Jung S, Abraham A, Gerlitz O, Pashut-Lavon I, Ben-Neriah Y (1995) *In vitro* stimulation of IκB phosphorylation is not sufficient to activate NF-κB. *Mol Cell Biol* 15: 1294–1301

88   DiDonato JA, Mercurio F, Karin M (1995) Phosphorylation of IκBα precedes but is not sufficient for its dissociation from NF-κB. *Mol Cell Biol* 15: 1302–1311

89   Traenckner EB-M, Wilk S, Baeuerle PA (1994) A proteasome inhibitor prevents activa-tion of NF-κB and stabilizes a newly phosphorylated form of IκB-α that is still bound to NF-κB. *EMBO J* 13: 5433–5441

90   Alkalay I, Yaron A, Hatsubai A, Orian A, Ciechanover A, Ben-Neriah Y (1995) Stimu-lation-dependent IκBα phosphorylation marks the NF-κB inhibitor for degradation via the ubiquitin-proteasome pathway. *Proc Natl Acad Sci USA* 92: 10599–10603

91   Li C-CH, Dai RM, Longo DL (1995) Inactivation of NF-κB inhibitors IκBα: ubiquitin-dependent proteolysis and its degradation product. *Biochem Biophys Res Comm* 213: 293–301

92   Baldi L, Brown K, Franzoso G, Siebenlist U (1996) Critical role for lysines 21 and 22 in signal-induced ubiquitin-mediated proteolysis of IκB-α. *J Biol Chem* 271: 376–379

93   Yaron A, Gonen H, Alkalay I, Hatzubai A, Jung S, Beyth S, Mercurio F, Manning AM, Ciechanover A, Ben-Neriah Y (1998) Inhibition of NF-κB cellular function via specific targeting of the IκB-ubiquitin ligase. *EMBO J* 16: 6486–6494

94   Palombella VJ, Rando OJ, Goldberg AL, Maniatis T (1994) The ubiquitin-proteasome pathway is required for processing the NF-κB1 precursor protein and the activation of NF-κB. *Cell* 78: 773–785

95   Lin Y-Z, Yao S, Veach RA, Torgerson TR, Hawiger J (1995) Inhibition of nuclear translocation of transcription factor NF-κB by a synthetic peptide containing a cell membrane-permeable motif and nuclear localization sequence. *J Biol Chem* 270: 14255–14258

Small molecule regulators of AP-1 and NF-κB

Anthony M. Manning

Signal Pharmaceuticals, Inc., 5555 Oberlin Drive, San Diego, CA 92121, USA

Introduction

Activator protein-1 (AP-1) is a pivotal transcription factor which regulates T-cell activation, cytokine production, and production of matrix metalloproteinases [1]. AP-1 includes members of the Jun and Fos families of transcription factors, which are characterized by basic region-leucine zipper (bZIP) DNA-binding domains. AP-1 proteins bind to DNA and activate transcription as Jun homodimers, Jun-Jun heterodimers, or Jun-Fos heterodimers. There are multiple Jun and Fos family members (c-Jun, JunB, JunD and c-Fos, FosB, Fra-1, Fra-2) which are expressed in different cell types and mediate the transcription of both unique and overlapping genes. AP-1 is also a component of the nuclear factor of activated T cells (NFAT) complex responsible for the transcription of the IL-2 gene and other cytokine genes in activated T cells [2].

MAPK pathways regulate the transcriptional activity of AP-1, both at the level of *de novo* synthesis of AP-1 family proteins and by controlling their transactivation function (Fig. 1) [3–6]. MAPK cascades consist of three- or four-tiered signaling modules in which the MAPK is activated by a MAP kinase kinase (MAPKK), which in turn is activated by a MAP kinase kinase kinase (MAPKKK) (Fig. 1). The MAPKKK is itself activated by a small G protein such as Ras, either directly or *via* another upstream kinase [7]. Three such MAPK signaling cascades, culminating in activation of the ERK, JNK and p38 MAP families of MAPK have been investigated in detail. The JNKs and p38 kinases are activated in response to the pro-inflammatory cytokines TNFα and IL-1, and by cellular stress (e.g. heat shock, osmotic shock, reactive oxygen metabolites, protein synthesis inhibitors, UV irradiation). The MAPKs are proline-directed serine/threonine kinases, which are activated by phosphorylation on closely-spaced threonine and tyrosine residues within the activation loop; the activation sequences characteristic of the ERK, JNK and p38 MAP kinase families are TEY, TPY, and TGY, respectively. These sequences are targets for phos-

Inflammatory Processes: Molecular Mechanisms and Therapeutic Opportunities, edited by L. Gordon Letts and Douglas W. Morgan
© 2000 Birkhäuser Verlag Basel/Switzerland

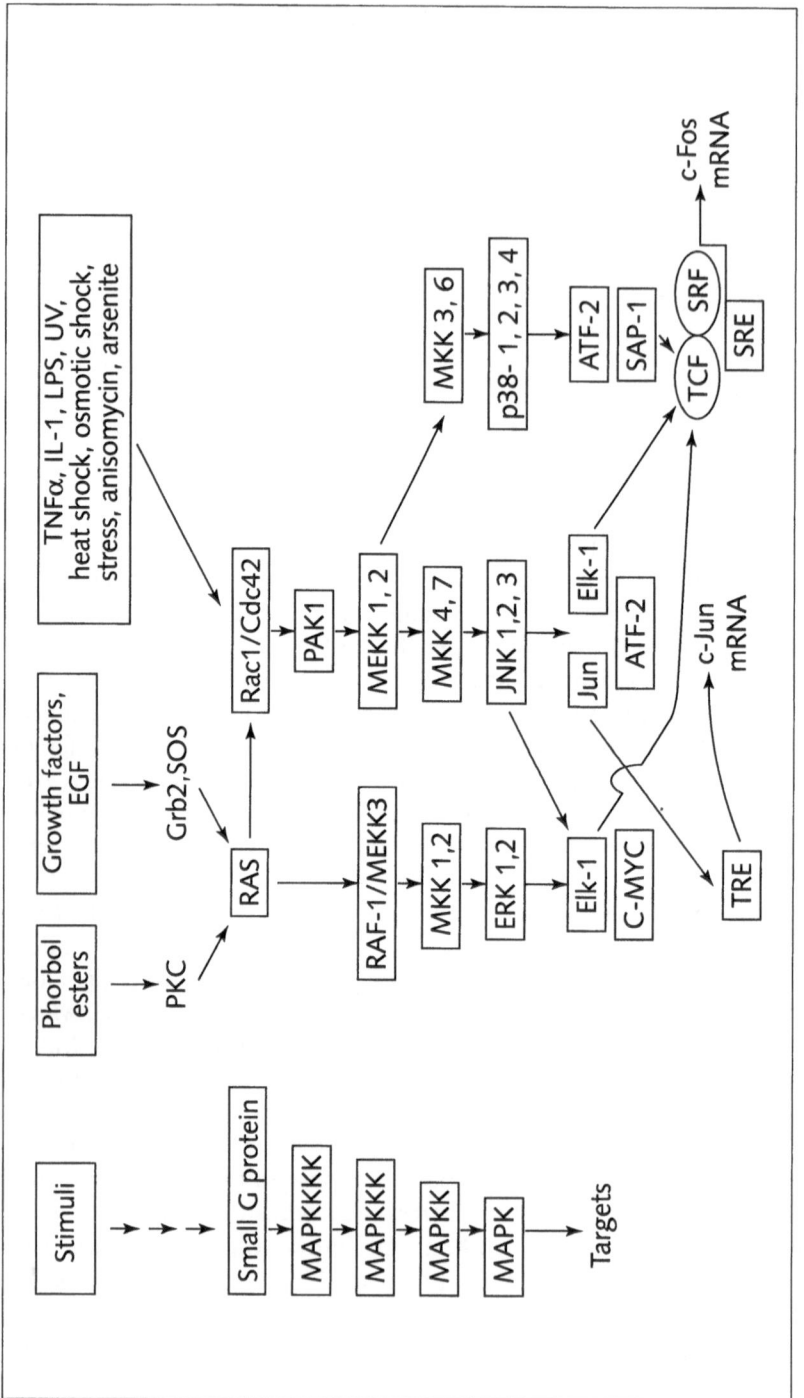

Figure 1

MAP kinase regulation of AP-1. Extracellular stimuli activate the ERK, JNK and p38 MAPK pathways through Ras and Rac-mediated processes. The ERK, JNK and p38 MAPKs phosphorylate the Elk-1 and SAP-1a transcription factors, resulting in enhanced c-Jun and c-Fos transcription and protein production. In addition, JNK 1, 2 and 3 phosphorylate the Jun subunit of AP-1 and directly enhance AP-1 transcactivating potential.

phorylation by specific MAPKKs, dual specificity threonine/tyrosine kinases which are themselves activated by MAPKKK-mediated phosphorylation at a pair of serine residues in the activation loop [3, 4, 7].

While there is some cross-talk between the major MAPK pathways, cells maintain exquisite specificity with extracellular signals only activating their proper targets. This is a result of several factors that include preferred interactions between kinases within a module and between MAPKs and their substrates [8]. Recently, scaffold proteins that bind multiple components of the signaling cascade have been described. For example, JIP-1 (JNK-interacting protein-1) first characterized as a cytoplasmic inhibitor of the JNK pathway has been shown to selectively bind the MAPK module, MLK → MKK7 → JNK [5, 9]. It has no binding affinity for a variety of other MAPK cascade enzymes. Different scaffold proteins are likely to exist for other MAPK signaling cascades to preserve substrate specificity. Many of the studies that have reported cross-talks between the different pathways have employed over-expression of members of the signaling cascades. This often leads to the erroneous conclusion that no fidelity exists between the cascades.

All three MAPK pathways are involved in the transcriptional regulation of Fos- and Jun-family genes. The ERKs, JNKs, and p38 MAPKs each contribute to upregulation of c-Fos gene transcription, by phosphorylating and activating the Ets-family transcription factors Elk-1 and SAP-1 [10]. A major component of AP-1 regulation is a consequence of post translational modification; for example, c-Jun is regulated by phosphorylation at two N-terminal serines in the transactivation domain (amino acids 63 and 73). This is accomplished by the c-Jun N-terminal kinases JNK1 and JNK2, although JNK2 binds c-Jun with a 10-fold higher affinity than JNK1 [11]. and may be the physiologically relevant activator of AP-1.

The JNKs are encoded by three genes: JNK1, JNK2 and JNK3. JNK1 and JNK2 are ubiquitously expressed whereas JNK3 is selectively expressed in the brain, heart and testis [8]. Gene transcripts are alternatively spliced to produce four-JNK1 isoforms, four-JNK2 isoforms and two-JNK3 isoforms. Inhibitors of JNK-mediated AP-1 activation may prove to be novel anti-inflammatory/immunosuppressive agents that will inhibit inducible expression of inflammatory genes, without affecting AP-1 mediated housekeeping functions. In T cells JNK activation by co-stimulation through the antigen and CD28 receptors correlates with IL-2 induction [12]. Recently, the examination of JNK-deficient mice revealed that the JNK pathway is induced in Th1 cells (producers of IFNγ and TNFβ), but not in Th2 effector cells (producers of IL-4, IL-5, IL-6, IL-10 and IL-13) upon antigen stimulation [13]. Deletion of either JNK1 or JNK2 in mice resulted in a selective defect in the ability of Th1 effector cells to express IFNγ. This suggests that JNK1 and JNK2 do not have redundant functions in T cells and that they play different roles in the control of cell growth, differentiation and death. Mice with a homozygous disruption for the JNK3 gene are viable [14]. However, they are resistant to the excitotoxic stress response elicited by kainic acid, a glutamate receptor agonist. Kainic acid causes neuronal damage especially within the hippocampus. The neurotoxicity of kainic acid possibly results from the induction of c-Jun and increased AP-1 DNA binding activity. JNK3 inhibitors may be potentially useful in treating epilepsy and other neurodegenerative diseases such as stroke. Recently the x-ray crystal structure of the unphosphorylated form of JNK3 was reported and should provide assistance in designing selective JNK3 inhibitors [15]. JNK3 reveals similarities to the structures of cAMP-dependent protein kinase and ERK2 and p38.

AP-1 inhibitors

PD098059 (see Figs. 2a, 2b) was discovered in a biochemical screen for inhibitors of the ERK cascade [16]. PD098059 binds to the inactive form of MEK1, a primary MAPKK in the ERK cascade, with an IC50 of ~ 4 µM and blocks the phosphorylation required for MEK activation. Specificity of action was indicated by the inability of PD098059 to inhibit phosphorylation mediated by c-Raf, JNK, p38, PKA, PKC, v-Src, active MEK1 and several other serine/threonine and protein tyrosine kinases (including receptor tyrosine kinases). U0126 is another MEK inhibitor that was discovered in a cell-based screen for compounds which inhibited the activity of an AP-1-driven luciferase promoter-reporter construct [17]. U0126 has potent *in vitro* activity and blocks T-cell activation and proliferation in response to Con A or CD3 stimulation. In addition, this inhibitor demonstrated potent *in vivo* efficacy in models of inflammation and delayed type hypersensitivity. Of note, competition studies with radiolabelled compounds demonstrated that PD98059 and U0126 compete for a similar site on MEK that is distinct from the ATP or peptide substrate binding sites. Ro 09-2210, another inhibitor of MEK1, was recently reported [18]. This compound was identified during high throughput screening of microbial broths for inhibitors of anti-CD3 induced T-cell proliferation. Ro 09-2210 is a potent inhibitor of MEK1 (IC_{50} = 59 nM) and appears to function through a mechanism distinct from that of PD98059 and U0126.

While no specific JNK inhibitors have been described, isoform-specific inhibitors are being sought. The greatest attention and most progress has been made in the discovery of p38 MAPK inhibitors [19]. The important role of the p38 pathway in inflammatory processes resulted from studies using a series of pyridinyl imidazoles exemplified by SK&F 86002 and SB203580 [20]. These potent inhibitors of p38 activity block IL-1 and TNF production in lipopolysacharide stimulated human monocytes. SB 203580 competes with ATP for binding to p38 and is remarkably selective [21]. It does inhibit JNK2 but with a 10–20-fold lower potency than p38. SB 203580 binds p38 by inserting into the ATP-binding pocket. While the 4-fluorophenyl ring of the compound does not make contact with residues in the ATP-binding pocket it is in near proximity to the Thr 106 of the enzyme. Mutation of this amino acid to Met 106 makes p38 insensitive to SB 203580 [22]. Thr 106 is

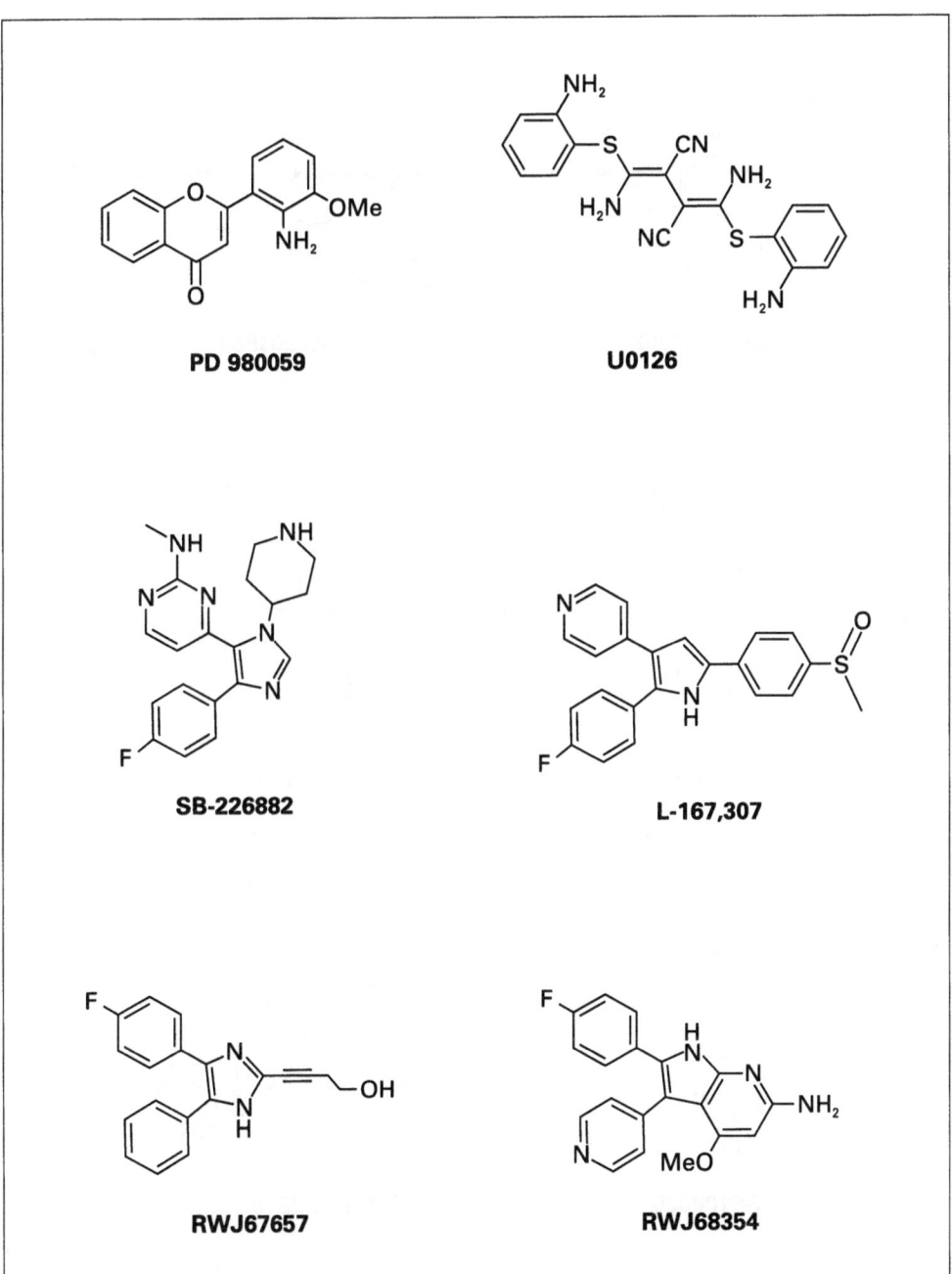

Figure 2a
Selected inhibitors of MAP kinases affecting AP-1.

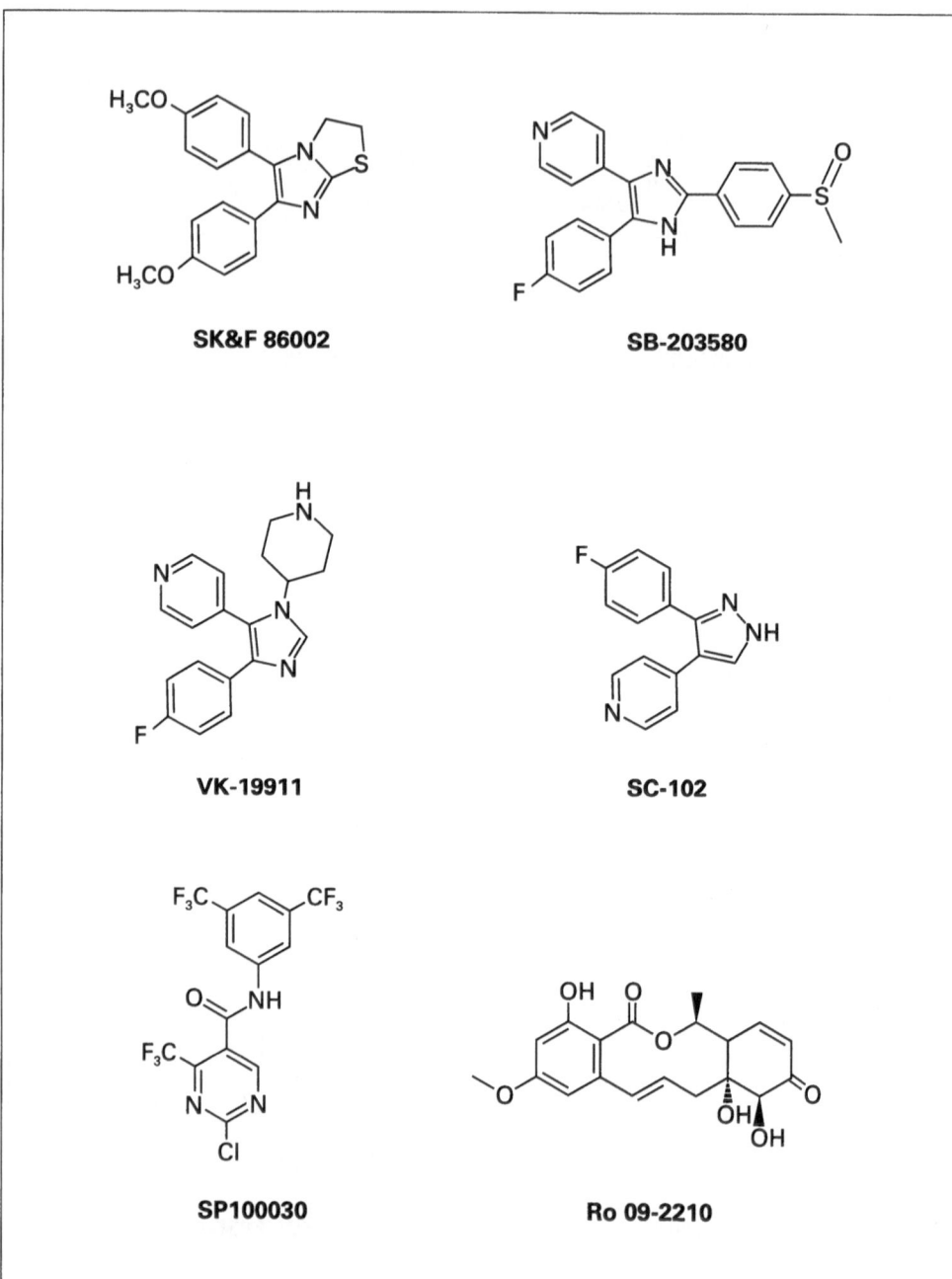

Figure 2b
Selected inhibitors of MAP kinases affecting AP-1.

conserved in p38β, another isoform of p38, that is sensitive to SB 203580, but is replaced by methionine in p38γ, p38δ, JNK1 and JNK2 (all much less sensitive to SB 203580). Mutation of p38β Thr106 to Met 106 rendered p38 almost resistant to SB 203580 and the reverse mutation of Met 106 to Thr106 in p38γ and p38δ resulted in SB 203580 sensitivity.

Some of the earlier p38 inhibitors, including SB 203580, are inhibitory towards several cytochrome p450 isoforms (1A2, 2C9, 2C19, 3A4, 2D6). This is due to the high-affinity binding of the 4-pyridyl group to heme iron. As a consequence, replacements for the 4-pyridyl ring were sought and the pyrimidine analog as represented by SB 226882 has equivalent p38 inhibitory potency in vitro and is effective in in vivo mouse models measuring circulating TNF levels. Several other p38 inhibitors have been reported including L-167, 307 [23], VK 19911 [24], and SC-102 RWJ 67657 and RWJ 68354 [25].

NF-κB pathways

Nuclear factor κB (NF-κB) was first described as a B cell-specific factor which bound to a short DNA sequence motif located in the immunoglobulin κ light chain enhancer, but it is now clear that NF-κB is expressed in all cell types and plays a broader role in gene transcription [26–28]. NF-κB plays a key role in the expression of as many as 70 genes central to the inflammatory response and has been detected in a variety of inflammatory settings in vivo including in atherosclerotic and restenotic lesions, in septicemia in humans, in rheumatoid synovium, and in UV-damaged skin [29]. NF-κB exists in the cytoplasm in an inactive form associated with inhibitory proteins termed IκB, of which the most important may be IκBα, IκBβ, and IκBε. Activation is achieved through the signal-induced proteolytic degradation of IκB in the cytoplasm.

Extracellular stimuli initiate a signaling cascade leading to activation of two IκB kinases, IKK-1 (IKKα) and IKK-2 (IKKβ) which phosphorylate IκB at specific N-terminal serine residues (S32 and S36 for IκBα, S19 and S23 for IκBβ) (Fig. 3) [30–33]. Phosphorylated IκB is then selectively ubiquinated, by an E3 ubiquitin ligase, the terminal member of a cascade of ubiquitin-conjugating enzymes. In the last step of this signaling cascade, phosphorylated and ubiquinated IκB, which is still associated with NF-κB in the cytoplasm, is selectively degraded by the 26S proteasome [34]. This process exposes the nuclear localization sequence (NLS), thereby freeing NF-κB to interact with the nuclear import machinery and translocate the nucleus, where it binds its target to initiate transcription.

The IκB kinases IKK-1 and IKK-2 are related members of a new family of intracellular signal transduction enzymes, containing an amino-terminal kinase domain and a C-terminal region with two protein interaction motifs, a leucine zipper and a helix-loop motif. There is strong evidence that IKK-1 and IKK-2 are themselves

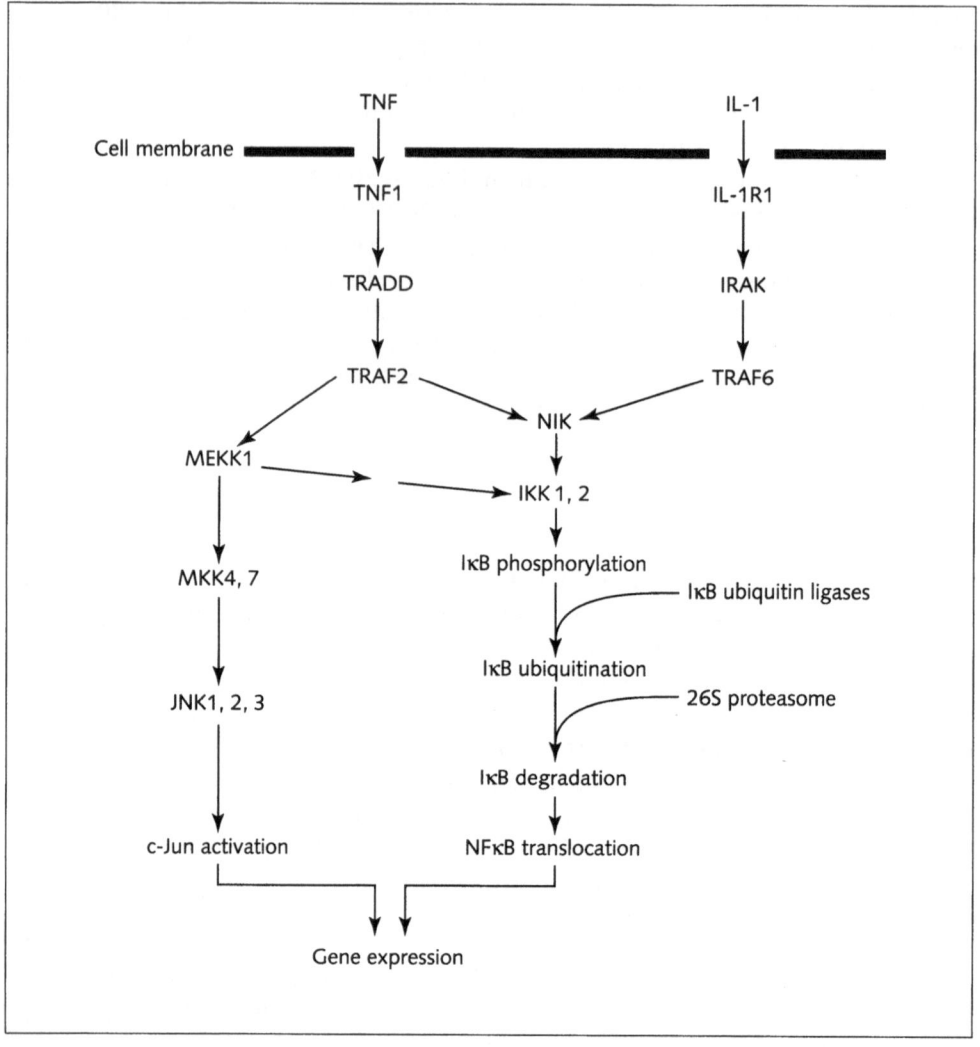

Figure 3
Signal transduction pathway regulating NF-κB activation by TNFα and IL-1. Activation of the TNF receptor type 1 (TNFR1) leads to recruitment of the TNF-receptor associated proteins TRADD and TRAF2, resulting in activation of the MAPK kinase kinases MEKK1 and NIK. Both these kinases have been implicated in the activation of the IκB kinases IKK1 and IKK2. NIK is also activated by IL-1 through the IL-1 recpetor associated kinase IRAK and TRAF6. Phosphorylation of the cytoplasmic inhibitor of NF-κB, IκB, leads to its ubiquitination and protelytic degradation by components of the ubiquitin-proteasome system. Free NF-κB within the cytoplasm is rapidly translocated to the nucleus where it modulates gene transcription.

phosphorylated and activated by one or more upstream activating kinases, which are likely to be members of the MAPKKK family of enzymes [32, 33]. NF-κB inducing kinase (NIK) was identified by its ability to bind directly to TRAF2, an adapter protein thought to couple both TNFα and IL-1 receptors to NF-κB [35]. A second MAPKKK, MEKK-1, was shown to be present in the IKK signalsome complex [32, 36].

Recently, we isolated the pIκBα-ubiquitin ligase from HeLa cells, through its specific association with the pIκBα/NF-κB complex [37]. The small polypeptide ubiquitin is transferred to specific proteins *via* a cascade of ligases that catalyze covalent attachment of ubiquitin to proteins. It appears there are only a small number of E1 ubiquitin ligases, and that specificity of ubiquitin transfer is mediated in large part by specific combinations of E2 and E3 ubiquitin ligases. In some cases, the E3 ligase does not directly transfer ubiquitin, but simply acts to mediate interaction of a specific protein substrate with an E2 ligase charged with ubiquitin. We initially purified an activity capable of specifically phosphorylating IκB in the presence of purified E1 and partially-purified E3 ligases from HeLa cells. This protein was identified as Ubc5c, an E2 ubiquitin ligase. The exquisite specificity of this system was demonstrated by the inability of Ubc5b, a related family member with approximately 90% sequence identity to Ubc5c, to re-constitute IκB ubiquitination *in vitro*. Using recombiannt NF-κB:IκB complexes, we purified two proteins which specifically bound when IκB was phosphorylated by IKK2. Nanoelectrospray mass spectrometry identified these polypeptides as two versions of the same protein and belonging to the recently identified β-TrCP/Slimb family. These proteins contain F box and WD domains, known to be involved in protein:protein interactions. The IκB-specific F box/WD protein bound specifically to pIκBα and promoted its ubiquitination in the presence of an E1 and Ubc5c, the IκB-specific E2 ubiquitin ligase. We therefore designated this IκB E3 ligase the E3 receptor subunit specific for IκBα, or E3RS[IκB]. A truncated version of this protein, containing only the F box IκB recognition motif, acted as a dominant negative molecule, inhibiting IκBα degradation and NF-κB activation in HeLa cells.

In addition to the IKKs and IκB ubiquitin ligase, there are additional kinase targets associated with the upstream activation of NF-κB [38]. Receptor-interacting protein (RIP) is a part of the TNF-receptor (TNF-R1) associated signaling complex along with TRADD and TRAF2. RIP is a serine/threonine kinase and the only component of the TNF-R1 signaling complex with enzymatic activity. However, no substrates have been identified for RIP. Analogous signaling components exist for the IL-1 receptor, they include IRAK, which is also a serine/threonine kinase that is autophosphorylated upon receptor activation. IRAK associates with TRAF6 to activate NF-κB; however, recombinant IRAK has no kinase activity. IKK-1 and IKK-2, their upstream activating kinases MEKK and NIK, and their downstream effector, the E3 ligase, all represent attractive targets for the discovery of drugs which selectively regulate NF-κB function.

NF-κB inhibitors

There are multiple targets that are amenable to small molecular blockade within the NF-κB activation pathway. No specific inhibitors of the enzymes mentioned above have been described. However, several NF-κB blockers have been reported and are reviewed elsewhere [27, 39]. Antioxidants and free radical scavengers such as N-acetylcysteine, curcumin and caffeic acid block NF-κB activation. The 26S proteasome contains a chymotrypsin-like activity that degrades IκB, an activity that can be blocked by peptide aldehydes including MG115, MG341 and Z-LLF-CHO [40, 41]. Several clinically important anti-inflammatory drugs such as salicylates, gold and glucocorticoids also inhibit NF-κB induced gene expression. Indeed, salicylates have recently been demonstrated to be specific inhibitors of IKK2 and to block IκB posphorylation and degradation [42]. Glucocorticoids may exert some of their anti-inflammatory effects by inducing the synthesis of IκB [43].

NF-κB and AP-1 inhibitors

A novel class of T-cell-specific inhibitors of NF-κB and AP-1 activity was recently identified in a cell-based screening effort to identify modulators of inflammatory gene expression [44, 45]. The most potent inhibitor in this series, SP100030, inhibits NF-κB- and AP-1-dependent reporter gene expression in stably-transfected Jurkat T cells with an IC_{50} of 30 nM. In stimulated Jurkat T cells, SP100030 inhibited the induced transcription of the IL-2, IL-8, TNFα and GM-CSF genes with a similar IC_{50}. The effects of SP100030 were specific for human T cells, demonstrating activity in four separate T-cell lines and in primary T cells isolated from whole human blood. SP100030 displayed no activity in non-T-cell lines, including monocytes, epithelial cells, fibroblasts, synoviocytes, osteoblasts and endothelial cells. SP100030 demonstrated efficacy in preclinical models of autoimmune disease, including adjuvant-induced arthritis, delayed type hypersensitivity, inflammatory bowel disease and allograft rejection [46]. SP100030 represents a new class of T-cell-specific dual inhibitors of NF-κB and AP-1 mediated inflammatory gene expression, and suggests that cell-specific inhibitors of inflammatory gene expression can indeed be identified. An interesting implication, possibly related to the cross-regulation of NF-κB and AP-1 activity by MAP kinase pathways, is that T cells possess a common target protein that controls the functions of both NF-κB and AP-1.

Future prospects

Because AP-1 and NF-κB are regulated by cascades of intracellular enzymes, including kinases and ubiquitin ligases, much of the current drug discovery efforts are focused on identifying specific inhibitors of these enzymes. Protein kinases play a key role in the regulation of AP-1 and NF-κB. While protein kinases are challenging drug targets the development of multiple kinase inhibitors for major clinical conditions is anticipated. Despite the conventional dogma that the catalytic site inhibitors are non-specific the identification of very selective kinase inhibitors has created considerable optimism for the future. In this age of increased chemical diversity it is anticipated that new kinase inhibitor templates will emerge from chemical and natural product libraries. For example, selective protein kinase inhibitors have recently been described based upon the unexpected binding of 2, 6, 9-trisubstituted purines to the ATP-binding site of human cyclin-dependent kinase 2 (CDK2) [47]. Such a combinatorial approach to modifying the purine scaffold creates an invaluable tool for identifying potentially selective kinase inhibitors. Natural products such as staurosporine and flavonoids such as quercetin and genistein have provided some of the earlier kinase inhibitor templates and will continue to be a valuable additional source of novel backbones. Finally, the rapid progress made in the production of crystal structures of a number of serine/threonine and tyrosine-specific protein kinases has identified the catalytic core of these important enzymes. We now know that this core consists of a small N-terminal domain largely composed of an antiparallel β-sheet, and a large C-terminal domain which is mostly α-helical. ATP is bound in the deep cleft that exists between both lobes and exposes its phosphate groups to the opening of the cleft where the substrate also binds. Conserved residues of the C-terminal domain interact with the γ-phosphate of ATP and provide the catalytic machinery for the kinase reaction. Often these protein kinases are activated by phosphorylation of sites in an activation region near the opening of the cleft. As greater knowledge of active site inhibitors for p38 as well as other kinases emerges it is becoming clearer how to modify compounds to create greater potency and specificity [48, 49].

Since protein kinases are intracellular enzymes, issues related to cell penetration, selectivity and *in vivo* efficacy and safety remain the challenge for the medicinal chemist. Enhanced screening capacities resulting from high throughput screening as well as the availability of multiple recombinant human kinases has expedited selective kinase inhibitor identification. Since there are many kinases within the cell, rapid and broad profiling remains an important goal for determining the secondary and tertiary events that are modified by selective kinase inhibition. Gene and protein profiling technologies will be useful for identifying compounds that act to coordinately regulate inflammatory genes without influencing housekeeping functions. Such profiles will be extremely useful in the selection and optimization of drug candidates. Issues that remain unanswered include the preferred site for targeted intervention on the kinase cascades. Is it better to develop a MAPKKK inhibitor or a MAPK inhibitor, for example? Will inhibitors of IKK1 influence NF-κB activation in the same way inhibitors of IKK2 will? The coming years should yield answers to these questions.

References

1 Foletta VC, Segal DH, Cohen DR (1998) *J Leukoc Biol* 63: 139
2 Rao A, Luo C, Hogan PG (1997) *Ann Rev Immunol* 15: 707
3 Karin M, Hunter T (1999) *Curr Biol* 5: 747
4 Su B, Karin M (1996) *Curr Opin Immunol* 8: 402
5 Whitmarsh AJ, Cavanaugh J, Tournier C et al (1998) *Science* 281: 1671
6 Whitmarsh AJ, Davis RJ (1996) *J Molec Med* 74: 589
7 Fanger GR, Gerwins P, Widmann C et al (1997) *Curr Opin Genet Devel* 7: 67
8 Ipp YT, Davis RJ (1998) *Curr Biol* 10: 205
9 Dickens M, Rogers JS, Cavanagh J et al (1997) *Science* 277: 693
10 Whitmarsh AJ, Shore P, Sharrocks AD, Davis RJ (1995) *Science* 269: 403
11 Kallunki T, Su B, Tsigelny I et al (1994) *Genes Dev* 8: 2996
12 Su B, Jacinto E, Hibi M et al (1994) *Cell* 77: 727
13 Yang DD, Conze D, Whitmarsh AJ et al (1998) *Immunity* 9: 575
14 Yang D, Tournier C, Wysk M et al (1997) *Nature* 389: 865
15 Xie X, Gu Y, Fox T, Coll JT et al (1998) *Structure* 6: 983
16 Dudley DT, Pang L, Decker SJ et al (1995) *Proc Nat Acad Sci USA* 95: 7686
17 Favata MF, Horiuchi KY, Manos EJ et al (1998) *J Biol Chem* 273: 18623
18 Williams DH, Wilkinson SE, Purton T et al (1998) *Biochem* 37: 9579
19 Lee JC, Laydon JT, McDonnell PC et al (1994) *Nature* 372: 739
20 Badger AM, Bradbeer JN, Votta B et al (1996) *J Pharmacol Exp Ther* 279: 1453
21 Tong L, Pav S, White DM et al (1998) *Nature Struct Biol* 4: 311
22 Eyers PA, Craxton M, Morrice N et al (1998) *Chem Biol* 5: 321
23 De Losazto SE, Visco D, Agarwal L et al (1998) *J Bioinorg Med* 8: 2689
24 Wilson KP, McCaffery PG, Hsiao K et al (1997) *Chem Biol* 4: 423
25 Henry JR, Rupert KC, Dodd JH et al (1998) *J Med Chem* 41: 4196
26 May MJ, Ghosh S (1998) *Immunol Today* 19: 80
27 Baeuerle PA, Baichwal VR (1997) *Adv Immunol* 65: 111
28 Manning AM (1998) *Curr Opin Drug Disc & Dev* 1: 147–156
29 Manning AM, Anderson DC (1994) *Ann Rev Med Chem* 29: 235
30 Regnier H, Song H, Gao H et al (1997) *Cell* 90: 373
31 Didonato J, Hayakawa M, Rothwarf DM et al (1997) *Nature* 388: 853
32 Mercurio F, Zhu H, Murray BW et al (1997) *Science* 278: 860
33 Woronicz JD, Gao X, Cao Z et al (1997) *Science* 278: 866
34 Chen Z, Hagler J, Palombella VJ et al (1995) *Genes Dev* 9: 1586
35 Malinin NL, Boldin MP, Kovalenko AV, Wallach D (1997) *Nature* 385: 540
36 Lee FS, Hagler J, Chen ZJ, Maniatis T (1997) *Cell* 88: 1586
37 Yaron A, Hatzubai A, Lavon I, Davis M, Amit S, Manning AM, Andersen JS, Mann M, Mercurio F, Ben-Neriah Y (1998) *Nature* 396: 590–594
38 Baichwal VJ, Baeuerle PA (1998) *Ann Rept Med Chem* 33: 233
39 Manning AM, Mercurio F (1997) *Exp Opin Invest Drugs* 6 (5): 1–13

40 Palombella VJ, Rando OL, Goldberg AL, Maniatis T (1994) *Cell* 78: 773

41 Traenckner B-ME, Wilk S, Baeuerle PA (1995) *EMBO J* 13: 5433

42 Min M-Y, Yamamoto Y, Gaynor R (1998) *Nature* 396: 77–80

43 Auphan N, DiDonato JA, Rosette C, Helmberg A, Karin M (1995) *Science* 270: 286–290

44 Suto MJ, Ransone LJ (1997) *Curr Pharmaceut Des* 3: 515

45 Sullivan RW, Bigam CG, Erdman P et al (1998) *J Med Chem* 41: 413

46 Goldman ME, Ransone LJ, Anderson DW, Gaarde WA, Suto MJ, Sullivan RW, Short-house R, Morikawa M, Morris RE (1996) *Trans Proc* 28: 3106–3109

47 Gray NS, Wodicka L, Thunnissen WH et al (1998) *Science* 281: 533

48 Taylor SS, Radzio-Andzelm E (1994) *Structure* 2: 345

49 Hang JZ, Zhang F, Ebert D et al (1995) *Structure* 3: 299

Mammalian target of rapamycin: Immunosuppressive drugs offer new insights into cell growth regulation

Robert T. Abraham

Department of Pharmacology and Cancer Biology, Room C333B LSRC, Box 3813, DUMC, Durham, NC 27710, USA

Introduction

In this "enlightened" era of drug development, molecular targets are validated on the basis of their relevance to specific disease states, and screening assays are developed to identify small molecule- or peptide-derived modulators of the selected target's function. However, the more classical paradigm, in which the clinical application of new compounds frequently preceded detailed studies of their molecular mechanisms of action, has not been entirely abandoned. Relevant examples are the natural product immunosuppressive agents, cyclosporine A, FK506, and rapamycin. These drugs (cyclosporine A and FK506 in particular) had already made indelible marks on the clinical field of organ transplantation by the time that bench scientists had begun to unravel the molecular pharmacology underlying their effects on immune responses. Remarkably, the insights provided by basic investigations into the cellular mechanisms of action of the immunosuppressants have been as impressive as the results obtained with these drugs in the clinical arena. In each case, the availability of the immunosuppressant enabled investigators to uncover novel and largely unexpected pathways of intracellular signaling. Ongoing research using cyclosporine A, FK506, and rapamycin as pharmacologic probes continues to yield new information relevant to the clinical management of organ transplants, autoimmune diseases, inflammation, and even cancer.

The focus of this brief monograph will be on rapamycin, the latest member of the group to enter the clinic, and the compound whose intracellular target was most recently identified. Although we are a long way from a complete understanding of the mechanism of action of rapamycin, it is clear that this drug interferes with a cell growth-related signal transduction pathway that has been fundamentally conserved during eukaryotic evolution from yeast to man. As stated above, the recent progress toward the definition of this signaling pathway is due in large part to the availabil-

Inflammatory Processes: Molecular Mechanisms and Therapeutic Opportunities, edited by L. Gordon Letts and Douglas W. Morgan
© 2000 Birkhäuser Verlag Basel/Switzerland

ity of the highly specific inhibitor, rapamycin. The results to date have provided at least a partial molecular explanation for the decades-old observation that cell growth is most sensitive to inhibitors of protein synthesis during G_1 phase of the cell cycle [1]. From a therapeutic viewpoint, rapamycin may prove to be the first member of a very unique class of immunosuppressive and anticancer agents targeted against growth-regulatory proteins whose expression is controlled at the level of translation. For reasons that continue to elude cell biologists, the passage of immunocompetent, proinflammatory, and certain tumor cells through G_1 phase is particularly sensitive to disruption of the translational control pathway governed by the rapamycin target protein, mTOR.

Pharmacology of rapamycin

Rapamycin is a macrolide ester produced by a bacterial strain that was cultured from a soil sample collected during a search for novel antibiotics in the Easter Islands. The pharmacologic basis of rapamycin's cellular actions has been reviewed in detail [2], and will be summarized briefly in this monograph. The structures of rapamycin and the related compound, FK506, are shown in Figure 1. Rapamycin is a hydrophobic macrolide ester that binds to a highly conserved and ubiquitously expressed cytoplasmic receptor termed FK506-binding protein-12 (FKBP12). The resulting FKBP12•rapamycin complex acquires an activity not expressed by either component of the complex in isolation, i.e. the ability to bind to and inhibit the kinase activities of specific target proteins termed, appropriately enough, target of rapamycin, or TOR proteins. Several aspects of this pharmacologic mechanism of action are worthy of special mention. First, rapamycin shares a common receptor, FKBP12, with the structurally related immunosuppressive agent, FK506. Moreover, the binding of FK506 to FKBP12 also represents an activation step leading to the formation of a proximate enzyme inhibitor. However, the similarity stops here, in that the FKBP12•FK506 complex targets a completely different signaling molecule, the Ca^{2+}-regulated serine-threonine phosphatase, calcineurin. This phosphatase is neither recognized nor inhibited by the FKBP12•rapamycin complex, and the converse is true as well – TOR protein function is unaffected by treatment of cells with FK506. Indeed, the drugs may be considered as mutual antagonists, because concomitant exposure of cells to FK506 and rapamycin may set up a competition for a limiting amount of the FKBP12 receptor protein. From the drug development viewpoint, the mechanism of action of rapamycin represents a fascinating solution to the daunting task of designing a small molecule inhibitor bearing a high level of specificity for a large polypeptide target. The FKBP12 receptor not only positions rapamycin in the optimal orientation to interact with the TOR proteins, but also supplies structural determinants that contribute to the affinity and specificity of this interaction.

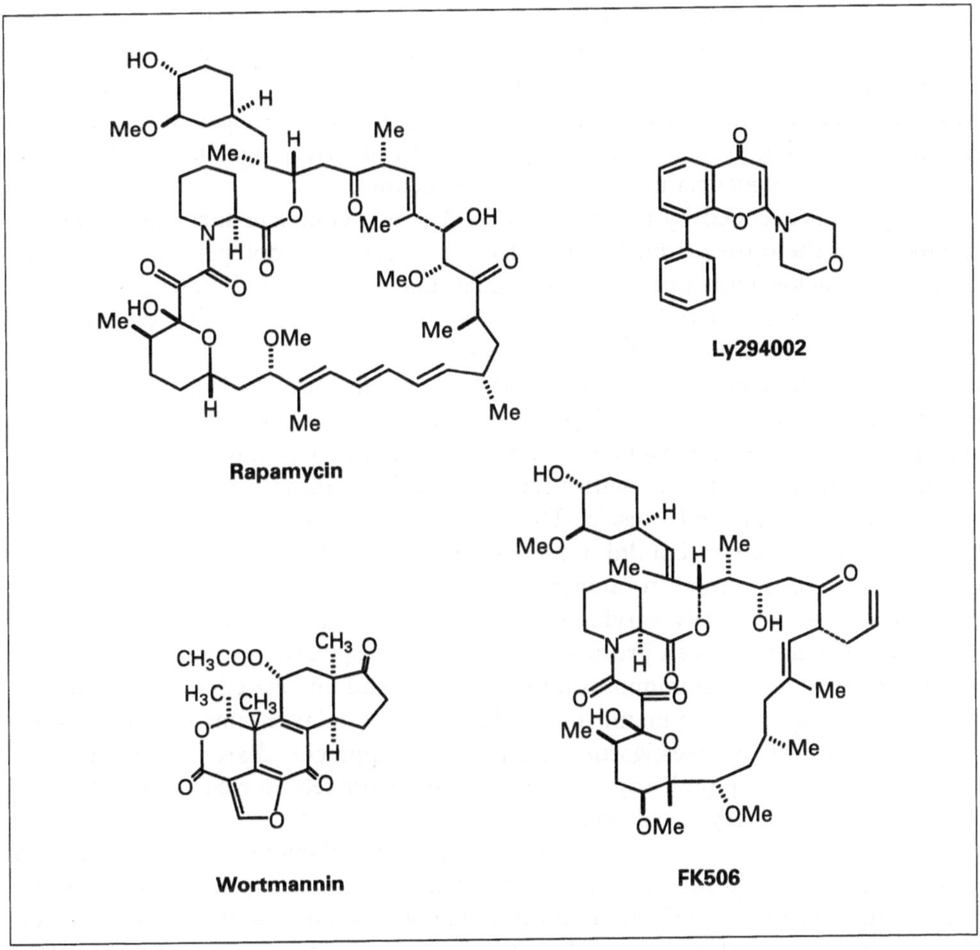

Figure 1
Structures of the macrolide immunosuppressants, FK506 and rapamycin, and the PI3K inhibitors, wortmannin and LY29002. Wortmannin binds irreversibly to and inhibits the catalytic activities of PI3Ks and many PIKKs, while the bioflavonoid derivative reversibly inhibits the catalytic activities of certain PI3Ks and PIKKs, including mTOR.

Identification of the rapamycin target protein

The strategy for the isolation of the rapamycin target protein was predicated on earlier work that led to the identification of calcineurin as the common ligand for the immunosuppressive complexes formed between FKBP12 and FK506, and cyclophilin A and cyclosporine A [3]. Mammalian tissue extracts were fractionated

55

to varying degrees, and then were passed over an affinity column containing FKBP12 loaded with rapamycin. Protein microsequence analysis led to the isolation of the full-length cDNA encoding the FKBP12•rapamycin-binding protein, which was named FRAP [4], RAFT1 [5], or mTOR [6] by the different laboratories. We termed this binding protein mammalian target of rapamycin (mTOR), in deference to the precedent nomenclature from yeast (see below).

The protein encoded by the mTOR cDNA was a complete surprise on several counts. First, the open reading frame encoded a very large polypeptide containing 2,549 amino acids, with a predicted molecular mass of 289 kilodaltons. Second, the only recognizable region of homology to other mammalian proteins resided near the carboxyl-terminus, which contained a stretch of approximately 400 amino acids that bore a distant but significant resemblance to the catalytic domains of phosphoinositide (PI) kinases, particularly those of PI 3-kinases (PI3Ks). Finally, the target protein, like the rapamycin receptor, FKBP12, was ubiquitously expressed in mammalian tissues and cells, with very high levels found in non-proliferating tissues, including brain and muscle. The latter results seemed in conflict with the observations that rapamycin did not behave like a broad-spectrum inhibitor of cell growth when administered to animals or humans. As stated above, a satisfactory explanation for the widely varying sensitivities of different tissue and cell types to rapamycin has not yet been proffered. What was recognized very quickly was that mechanistic studies of an immunosuppressive drug had uncovered a novel regulator of G_1 phase progression in mammalian cells. The molecular cloning of mTOR drew the attention of many investigators to a largely unappreciated area of signal transduction – the coupling pathway between growth factor receptor occupancy and the translational machinery in eukaryotic cells.

The deduced amino acid sequence of mTOR also told mammalian cell biologists that, as frequently has been the case in the signaling field, the yeast geneticists had "beaten them to the punch". In addition to its potent immunosuppressive activities, rapamycin is a powerful antifungal agent. Genetic screens for mutations that rendered the budding yeast, *Saccharomyces cerevesiae*, resistant to rapamycin yielded one known and two novel genes [7–9]. Mutations in the previously identified *FKP1* gene, which encodes the yeast FKBP12 ortholog, caused loss of rapamycin sensitivity. This resistant phenotype would be predicted on the basis of the pharmacology outlined above, as both FKBP12 and rapamycin are required for the cellular effects of the immunosuppressive drug. In addition, the screen revealed that mutations in either of two novel and highly related genes, *TOR1* and *TOR2*, permitted yeast cells to form colonies when plated onto a rapamycin-containing semisolid matrix. Remarkably, the sequences of the two yeast proteins exhibited greater than 40% overall identity to that of mTOR, and this sequence identity between the yeast and mammalian TORs rose to greater than 65% in the carboxyl-terminal region containing the PI3K-related catalytic domain. Clearly, TOR1p and TOR2p were orthologs of the subsequently identified mTOR polypeptide. When considered in light of the observation that rapamycin treatment arrests the growth of yeast cells in G_1 phase of the cell cycle, it became evident that the TOR proteins participated in a cell-cycle regulatory pathway that had been fundamentally conserved during the evolution of eukaryotic cells.

Additional genetic studies in S. *cerevesiae* demonstrated that the *TOR2* gene was essential for viability, while the *TOR1* gene was nonessential, although loss of *TOR1* caused yeast cells to grow more slowly in nutritious medium [10, 11]. Interestingly, a double disruption of the *TOR1* and *TOR2* genes resulted in G_1-phase growth arrest and gradual loss of viability – a phenotype that strongly resembled the response of wild-type yeast cells to rapamycin exposure. These results further solidified the argument that rapamycin exerted its cellular effects by inducing loss of a critical signaling function(s) of TOR1p and TOR2p in G_1-phase yeast cells.

Biochemical insights into the mechanicsm of action of rapamycin

The identification of mutant TOR1p and TOR2p polypeptides that led to rapamycin resistance in yeast provided valuable clues regarding the nature of the interaction of the TOR proteins with the FKBP12•rapamycin complex. The "hot spot" for the generation of biologically active but drug-resistant TOR proteins was a conserved serine residue in TOR1p and TOR2p that, when substituted by a more bulky amino acid (e.g. arginine or isoleucine), rendered the host cells resistant to rapamycin [7, 12–14]. We now know that this critical serine residue, which is also found in the mammalian ortholog, mTOR, is nested within a ~ 100 amino acid stretch of amino acids termed the FKBP12•rapamycin binding (FRB) domain [13, 14] (see Fig. 2). Interestingly, the FRB domain is located immediately upstream of the catalytic domain, and has no identifiable role in catalysis. Nonetheless, the interaction of this domain with the FKBP12•rapamycin complex strongly inhibits the kinase activity of mTOR. Although the mechanism remains unclear, a speculative proposal is that the bulky immunophilin•drug complex poses a steric hindrance to the presentation of protein substrates to the catalytic domain.

The findings described above highlight two pharmacological features that have greatly facilitated research concerning the signaling functions of mTOR in mammalian cells. First, rapamycin is an exquisitely specific inhibitor of mTOR function in intact cells; hence, any alteration in a cellular response induced by rapamycin strongly implicates a role for mTOR in the pathway leading to the response. Second, the availability of rapamycin-resistant, but otherwise fully functional, mTOR mutants permits detailed structure-function studies of this kinase in otherwise wild-type cells. Such mutants are readily generated by substitution of Ser[2035] in the FRB domain of mTOR with a more bulky substituent, such as Ile. The general strategy is then to introduce the rapamycin-resistant mTOR mutant into the appropriate cellular host, and then to treat these cells with rapamycin. The drug is assumed to

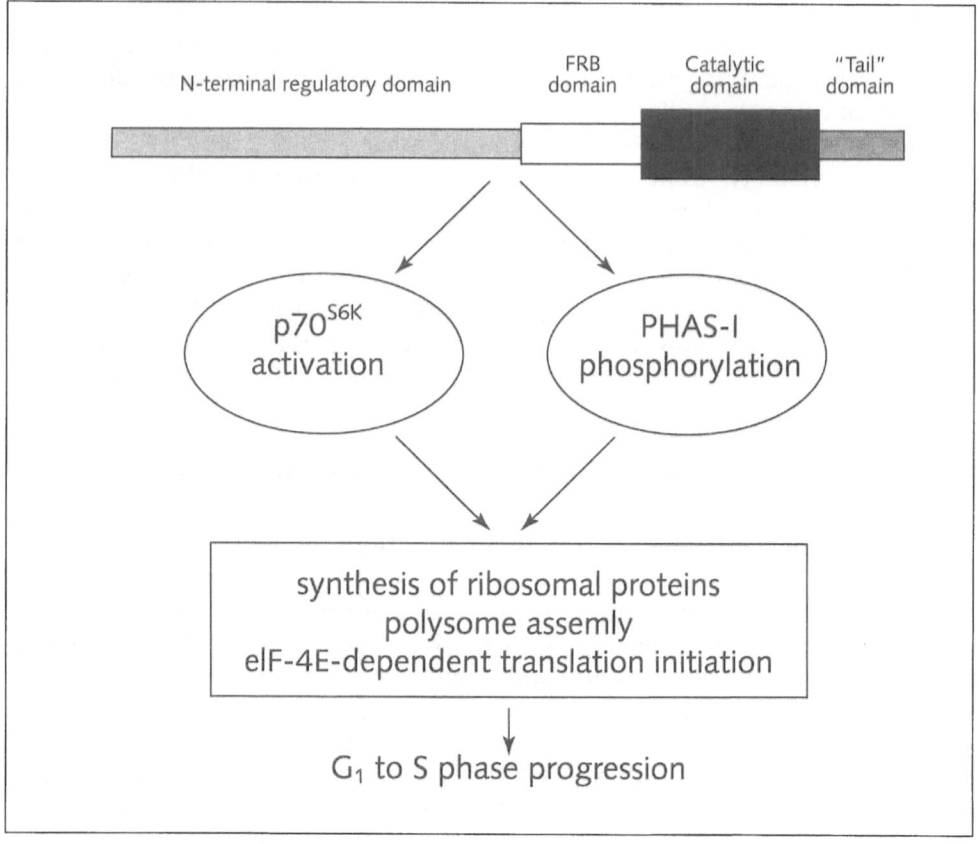

Figure 2
Structure and rapamycin-sensitive signaling functions of mTOR. The conceptual translation product of the mTOR cDNA is a 2,549 amino acid polypeptide containing a carboxyl-terminal region similar to the catalytic domains of PI3Ks. The function of the very extended N-terminal region (~ 1900 amino acids) is unclear, but this domain may play roles in protein-protein interactions and/or the subcellular localization of mTOR. The FRB domain comprises approximately 100 amino acids, and represents the binding site for the inhibitory FKBP12•rapamycin complex. The function of the "tail" domain, which contains approximately 30 amino acids, is also unclear, but deletion experiments indicate that this domain is essential for the protein kinase activity of mTOR.
The kinase activity of mTOR is required for the phosphorylation of p70^S6K and PHAS-I in mitogen-stimulated cells. Activation of p70^S6K facilitates the overall process of translation initiation, and specifically increases the synthesis of components of the protein synthesis machinery itself. The phosphorylation of PHAS-I leads to an increase in eIF-4E-dependent translation initiation, and may specifically augment the production of proteins required for G_1 to S phase progression.

effect a functional "knockout" of the rapamycin-sensitive functions of the endogenous mTOR proteins in these cells, thereby allowing one to focus on the signaling capabilities of the ectopically-expressed mTOR mutant. Although this approach has limitations, it has been instrumental in efforts to define the signaling functions of mTOR in mammalian cells.

A family of PI3K-related kinases

The months that followed the cloning of mTOR were marked by a flurry of activity leading to the identification of a large and still-growing family of signaling proteins that contain the PI3K-like catalytic domain. This novel family of proteins, which we term PI3K-related kinases (PIKKs), has been the subject of several reviews [15-17]. The PIKK family currently contains four mammalian proteins: mTOR, ataxia telangiectasia-mutated (ATM), ATM- and Rad3-related (ATR), and DNA-dependent protein kinase (DNA-PK). A mammalian cDNA encoding a Myc-interacting protein, termed TRRAP, may be the newest addition to the PIKK family [18]. However, the deduced sequence suggests that the region of similarity to the PI3K catalytic domain may not possess phosphotransferase activity. In contrast to the TOR proteins, the remaining members of the PIKK family appear not to be involved in the transmission of mitogenic signals from the cell surface. Rather, this subgroup of PIKKs, which includes ATM, ATR, and DNA-PK, participate in genome surveillance and maintenance by functioning as components of cell-cycle checkpoints and the DNA repair machinery. This subgroup has attracted considerable attention from cancer researchers, because a hallmark characteristic of cancer cells is genomic instability, a phenotype that can be traced to the breakdown of one or more cell-cycle checkpoints. The importance of cell-cycle checkpoints during normal development is underscored in dramatic fashion by the catastrophic consequences of the loss of ATM function in humans. AT patients exhibit chromosome instability leading to neurodegeneration, immunodeficiency, elevated cancer susceptibility, and hypersensitivity to radiation and other DNA-damaging agents. It is particularly noteworthy, that, at this early stage of our understanding, the PIKK family already holds a novel target (mTOR) for a clinically relevant immunosuppressant, and a checkpoint kinase (ATM) whose loss explains the complex phenotype of a long-studied human disease.

Effects of rapamycin on mammalian cell growth

One notable difference between yeast and mammalian cells is that the latter cells display widely varying sensitivities to the growth-inhibitory effect of rapamycin, depending on the cell lineage, as well as the growth factor milieu in which the response to the drug is being evaluated. Although the actual determinants of rapamycin sensitivity or resistance have not been defined, recent insights into the mTOR-dependent signaling pathway may eventually yield the answer to this crucial question (see below). A prototypical target cell for rapamycin is the activated T lymphocyte, which undergoes G_1 to S phase progression in response to IL-2 or T-cell growth-promoting cytokines. IL-2-stimulated T cells accumulate in mid/late G_1 phase of the cell cycle in the presence of ≤ 10 nM rapamycin [19, 20]. The growth-arrested T cells are characterized by the presence of fully assembled but catalytically inactive cyclin E-Cdk2 complexes, the maintenance of the under-phosphorylated, and hence growth-suppressive form of the retinoblastoma protein (pRb), in spite of continuous exposure to IL-2. Rapamycin treatment seems to allow T cells to progress up to the so-called G_1 restriction point, but does not permit passage through this important checkpoint. Restriction point traverse, which depends on the hyperphosphorylation, and inactivation of pRb marks the transition from growth factor-dependent cell-cycle progression to an intrinsic commitment of the cell-cycle machinery to execute S, G2, and M phases [1]. Thus, the rapamycin target, mTOR, must mediate the delivery of signals required for the progression of G_1-phase T cells through the restriction point.

Role of mTOR in translational control

The search for more proximal biochemical responses to rapamycin treatment led to the identification of two proteins whose phosphorylation state is regulated by mTOR. The first target protein is p70 S6 kinase (p70[S6K]), a serine-threonine kinase that is activated in response to a broad range of mitogenic stimuli. Rapamycin blocks both the phosphorylation and activation of p70[S6K] in all mammalian cell types examined to date. The second endpoint for the mTOR-dependent phosphorylation pathway is the translational-repressor protein, PHAS-I (also termed 4E-BP1) [21]. As mentioned above, it is striking that both p70[S6K] and PHAS-I participate in the regulation of protein synthesis in cells stimulated with mitogens or certain hormones, including insulin.

The regulation of p70[S6K] by upstream protein kinases is exceedingly complex, and the reader is referred to specialized reviews for details concerning this topic [22, 23]. However, it is clear that treatment with rapamycin quickly and efficiently inhibits the *de novo* phosphorylation of p70[S6K] induced by hormonal stimuli, as well as the phosphorylation of previously activated p70[S6K]. The predicted epistatic relationship between mTOR and p70[S6K] was confirmed in cell transfection experiments, which demonstrated that introduction of a rapamycin-resistant mTOR mutant into Jurkat T cells rendered p70[S6K] activation correspondingly resistant to rapamycin [24]. The only documented physiologic substrate for p70[S6K] is the 40S ribosomal protein S6, although recent data suggest that this protein kinase also phosphorylates two translation initiation factors, eIF-4G and eIF-4B [25]. The overall effect of these phosphorylation events is to increase the capacity of the protein synthetic machinery to translate mRNA templates. This modulation of translational capacity is logical, when one considers that successful passage through G_1 requires a substantial increase in cell mass, if the mitotic cycle is destined to give rise to two normally sized daughter cells.

Regulation of translation initiation by mTOR

The rate-limiting step in the translation of most eukaryotic mRNAs is initiation, a process that includes the binding of the 43S ribosomal preinitiation complex to the 5'-terminus of the mRNA, and the 5'→3' translocation of this complex as it scans the 5'-UTR for an AUG initiation codon [25, 26]. Both the ribosome binding and scanning steps are facilitated by the eukaryotic initiation factor (eIF)-4F complex, which itself binds to the cap structure (m^7GpppN, where N is any nucleotide) found at the extreme 5'-terminus of nearly all eukaryotic mRNAs. The eIF-4F complex contains eIF-4G, a large scaffolding protein, eIF-4A, an ATP-dependent RNA helicase (when partnered with an additional initiation factor, eIF-4B), and eIF-4E, the mRNA cap-binding subunit. An exciting realization over the past several years is that rates of translation initiation are controlled by extracellular stimuli, including growth factors, cytokines, and insulin. Moreover, this regulatory mechanism is highly discriminate: in mitogen-stimulated cells, translation of some mRNAs increases dramatically (> 30-fold) while the overall increase in protein synthesis is quite modest (1.5–2-fold).

The major determinants of eIF-4F dependence reside within the 5'-UTRs of translatable mRNAs. In quiescent cells, mRNAs bearing 5'-UTRs with extensive secondary structure and/or multiple upstream open reading frames tend to be translated very inefficiently due to impaired initiation. Interestingly, a number of growth-regulatory proteins (e.g. c-Myc, cyclin D_1 and ornithine decarboxylase) are encoded by mRNAs that contain such structural complexity in their 5'-UTRs. Mitogenic stimuli increase the translational efficiencies of these mRNAs by stimulating eIF-4F binding and function, often through the phosphorylation of specific components of this complex. Collectively, this "activated" eIF-4F increases both ribosome binding to the mRNA, and simplifies the structure of the 5'-UTR *via* the RNA-unwinding activity of eIF-4A, acting in concert with eIF-4B. The positive regulatory effect of mitogens on eIF-4F function therefore provides a mechanism by which the expression of certain growth-related genes can be controlled at the translational level.

The cap-binding eIF-4E subunit is a target for multiple intracellular signaling pathways, including the pathway governed by mTOR. The interaction of eIF-4E with the remaining components of the eIF-4F complex is competitively inhibited by the formation of complexes with 4E-binding proteins (4E-BPs) [21, 27]. These eIF-

4E interactors are also termed PHAS (phosphorylated heat and acid stable) proteins, and, for historical reasons, we will use the latter terminology for the remainder of this discussion. The most well-studied member of this family of eIF-4E inhibitors is PHAS-I. In quiescent cells, PHAS-I is not phosphorylated, and is tightly bound to eIF-4E. Under these conditions, eIF-4F function, and therefore translation initiation, is repressed. Exposure of these cells to growth factors or insulin results in the rapid phosphorylation of PHAS-I at 5 serine or threonine residues, and a consequent decrease in the binding affinity of PHAS-I for eIF-4E. Thus, the multi-site phosphorylation of PHAS-I removes a significant obstacle to eIF-4E-dependent translation initiation, and facilitates the synthesis of proteins needed for G_1-phase progression.

The protein kinase(s) responsible for the phosphorylation of PHAS-I quickly became a topic of considerable interest. A seminal observation was that this response was blocked by growth-inhibitory concentrations of rapamycin, which strongly hinted that mTOR served as an upstream kinase in the PHAS-I phosphorylation pathway [28–30]. In a somewhat unexpected turn of events, it was recently shown that mTOR itself phosphorylates PHAS-I, at least under *in vitro* kinase assay conditions [31]. The physiologic relevance of these findings is supported by the findings that the five sites phosphorylated by mTOR *in vitro* are identical to the sites of PHAS-I phosphorylation during insulin stimulation of intact cells [32, 33]. The same serine and threonine residues are rapidly dephosphorylated upon addition of rapamycin to these cells. Finally, the *in vitro* phosphorylation of PHAS-I by mTOR effectively inhibits the binding of PHAS-I to eIF-4E. Collectively, these findings argue that mTOR may be directly responsible for the phosphorylation of PHAS-I and subsequent activation of eIF-4E induced by insulin and other mitogenic factors.

Regulation of mTOR activity by hormonal stimuli

An important area for ongoing studies concerns the pathways through which mTOR is regulated in response to extracellular stimuli. Signals emanating from activated PI3K have been implicated in the stimulation of protein synthesis for some time. More recent evidence suggests that both PI3K and its downstream serine-threonine kinase, AKT, participate in mTOR activation by insulin and other polypeptide hormones [34, 35]. Interestingly, the carboxyl-terminal region of mTOR contains at least two consensus sites for phosphorylation by AKT, and indirect evidence suggests that these sites are, in fact, phosphorylated in an AKT-dependent fashion in intact cells [35]. These findings also raise some cautionary points concerning the extensive laboratory application of wortmannin, an irreversible inhibitor of PI3K, as a signal transduction inhibitor in mammalian cells. Treatment of cells with wortmannin will interfere with at least two components of the cytokine receptor-linked pathway leading to translation initiation: the lipid kinase activity of the p85-p110 form of PI3K and, as reported recently, the protein kinase activity of mTOR [31]. Wortmannin irreversibly inhibits the PHAS-I phosphorylating activity of mTOR with an IC_{50} of 250 nM [36]. Although the potency of wortmannin as an mTOR kinase inhibitor is approximately 100-fold lower than that observed with p85-p110 as the target (IC_{50}, 3 nM), the emergence of mTOR and other members of the PIKK family [37] as wortmannin-sensitive kinases complicates the interpretation of results based on the use of this broad spectrum inhibitor of kinases containing the PI3K-related catalytic domain.

Summary and perspective

Rapamycin is a potent immunosuppressive drug that seems destined to find important applications in the transplantation clinic, and in the treatment of autoimmune disease and, possibly, certain types of cancer. Studies of the mechanism of action of rapamycin indicate that this drug blocks the growth of lymphoid and other cell types by suppressing the protein kinase activity of mTOR. The rapamycin target protein, mTOR, functions in a highly conserved signaling pathway leading to the activation of the translational enhancer, $p70^{S6K}$ and the functional inactivation of the translational repressor, PHAS-I. The mTOR signaling pathway seems to be required for the translation of certain mRNAs whose protein products carry out functions permissive for the passage of G_1-phase cells through the restriction point. The discovery that mTOR is a serine-threonine protein kinase should facilitate the further development of new drugs that, like rapamycin, interfere in a relatively subtle fashion with the biochemical pathway that links cytokine receptor occupancy to the synthesis of proteins involved in the control of cell growth.

From a broader perspective, the use of rapamycin as a pharmacologic probe opened an avenue of investigation that led to the identification of a completely novel family of signaling proteins, the PIKKs. Ongoing studies of the PIKKs will provide novel insights into the mechanisms whereby normal cells regulate their growth and maintain the integrity of their genomes. The information already available strongly suggests that PIKK dysfunction will lead to defects in the development of the nervous and immune systems, and will favor the development of cancer in humans. At the same time, however, members of the PIKK family have considerable potential as targets for the development of novel anticancer and immunosuppressive agents.

Acknolwedgements
The author wishes to thank Drs. Aleksander Sekulic and Christine Hudson for helpful discussions. Work performed in the author's laboratory was supported by a Admadjaja Thymoma Research Grant from the Mayo Foundation, and by a grant (CA76193) from the National Cancer Institute.

References

1   Pardee AB (1989) G_1 events and the regulation of cell proliferation. *Science* 246: 603–640

2   Abraham RT, Wiederrecht GJ (1996) Immunopharmacology of rapamycin. *Ann Rev Immunol* 14: 483–510

3   Schreiber SL, Crabtree GR (1992) The mechanism of action of cyclosporin A and FK506. *Immunol Today* 13: 136–142

4   Brown EJ, Albers MW, Shin TB, Ichikawa K, Keith CT, Lane WS, Schreiber SL (1994) A mammalian protein targeted by G_1-arresting rapamycin-receptor complex. *Nature* 369: 756–758

5   Sabatini DM, Erdjument-Bromage H, Lui M, Tempst P, Snyder SH (1994) RAFT1: a mammalian protein that binds to FKBP12 in a rapamycin-dependent fashion and is homologous to yeast TORs. *Cell* 78: 35–43.

6   Sabers CJ, Martin MM, Brunn GJ, Williams JM, Dumont FJ, Wiederrecht G, Abraham RT (1995) Isolation of a protein target of the FKBP12-rapamycin complex in mammalian cells. *J Biol Chem* 270: 815–822

7   Helliwell SB, Wagner P, Kunz J, Deuter-Reinhard M, Henriquez R, Hall MN (1994) TOR1 and TOR2 are structurally and functionally similar but not identical phosphatidylinositol kinase homologues in yeast. *Molec Biol Cell* 5: 105–118

8   Heitman J, Movva NR, Hall MN (1992) Proline isomerases at the crossroads of protein folding, signal transduction, and immunosuppression. *New Biologist* 4: 448–460

9   Cafferkey R, Young PR, McLaughlin MM, Bergsma DJ, Koltin Y, Sathe GM, Faucette L, Eng WK, Johnson RK, Livi GP (1993) Dominant missense mutations in a novel yeast protein related to mammalian phosphatidylinositol 3-kinase and VPS34 abrogate rapamycin cytotoxicity. *Mol Cell Biol* 13: 6012–6023

10 Kunz J, Henriquez R, Schneider U, Deuter-Reinhard M, Movva NR, Hall MN (1993) Target of rapamycin in yeast, TOR2, is an essential phosphatidylinositol kinase homolog required for G1 progression. *Cell* 73: 585–596

11 Zheng XF, Florentino D, Chen J, Crabtree GR, Schreiber SL (1995) TOR kinase domains are required for two distinct functions, only one of which is inhibited by rapamycin. *Cell* 82: 121–130

12 Stan R, McLaughlin MM, Cafferkey R, Johnson RK, Rosenberg M, Livi GP (1994) Interaction between FKBP12-rapamycin and TOR involves a conserved serine residue. *J Biol Chem* 269: 32027–32030

13 Chen J, Zheng XF, Brown EJ, Schreiber SL (1995) Identification of an 11-kDa FKBP12-rapamycin-binding domain within the 289-kDa FKBP12-rapamycin-associated protein and characterization of a critical serine residue. *Proc Natl Acad Sci USA* 92: 4947–4951

14 Lorenz MC, Heitman J (1995) TOR mutations confer rapamycin resistance by preventing interaction with FKBP12-rapamycin. *J Biol Chem* 270: 27531–27537

15 Keith CT, Schreiber SL (1995) PIK-related kinases: DNA repair, recombination, and cell cycle checkpoints. *Science* 270: 50–51

16 Abraham RT (1996) Phosphoinositide 3-kinase related kinases. *Curr Op Immunol* 8: 412–418

17 Hunter T (1995) When is a lipid kinase not a lipid kinase? When it is a protein kinase. *Cell* 83: 1–4

18 McMahon SB, Van Buskirk HA, Dugan KA, Copeland TD, Cole MD (1998) The novel ATM-related protein TRRAP is an essential cofactor for the c-Myc and E2F oncoproteins. *Cell* 94: 363–374

19 Morice WG, Brunn GJ, Wiederrecht G, Siekierka JJ, Abraham RT (1993) Rapamycin-induced inhibition of p34cdc2 kinase activation is associated with G1/S-phase growth arrest in T lymphocytes. *J Biol Chem* 268: 3734–3738

20 Morice WG, Wiederrecht G, Brunn GJ, Siekierka JJ, Abraham RT (1993) Rapamycin inhibition of interleukin-2-dependent p33cdk2 and p34cdc2 kinase activation in T lymphocytes. *J Biol Chem* 268: 22737–22745

21 Lawrence JC Jr, Abraham RT (1997) PHAS/4E-BPs as regulators of mRNA translation and cell proliferation. *Trends Biochem Sci* 22: 345–349

22 Proud CG (1996) p70 S6 kinase: an enigma with variations. *Trends Biochem Sci* 21: 181–185

23 Pullen N, Thomas G (1997) The modular phosphorylation and activation of p70s6k. *FEBS Lett* 410: 78–82

24 Brown EJ, Beal PA, Keith CT, Chen J, Shin TB, Schreiber SL (1995) Control of p70 s6 kinase by kinase activity of FRAP *in vivo*. *Nature* 377: 441–446

25 Sonenberg N, Gingras AC (1998) The mRNA 5' cap-binding protein eIF4E and control of cell growth. *Curr Op Cell Biol* 10: 268–275

26 Pain VM (1996) Initiation of protein synthesis in eukaryotic cells. *Eur J Biochem* 236: 747–771

27 Pause A, Belsham GJ, Gingras AC, Donze O, Lin TA, Lawrence JC Jr, Sonenberg N (1995) Insulin-dependent stimulation of protein synthesis by phosphorylation of a regulator of 5'-cap function. *Nature* 371: 762–767

28 Graves LM, Bornfeldt KE, Argast GM, Krebs EG, Kong X, Lin TA, Lawrence JC Jr (1995) cAMP- and rapamycin-sensitive regulation of the association of eukaryotic initiation factor 4E and the translational regulator PHAS-I in aortic smooth muscle cells. *Proc Natl Acad Sci USA* 92: 7222–7226

29 Lin TA, Kong X, Saltiel AR, Blackshear PJ, Lawrence JC Jr (1995) Control of PHAS-I by insulin in 3T3-L1 adipocytes. Synthesis, degradation, and phosphorylation by a rapamycin-sensitive and mitogen-activated protein kinase-independent pathway. *J Biol Chem* 270: 18531–18538

30 Beretta L, Gingras AC, Svitkin YV, Hall MN, Sonenberg N (1996) Rapamycin blocks the phosphorylation of 4E-BP1 and inhibits cap-dependent initiation of translation. *EMBO J* 15: 658–664

31 Brunn GJ, Hudson CC, Sekulic A, Williams JM, Hosoi H, Houghton PJ, Lawrence JC, Abraham RT (1997) Phosphorylation of the translational repressor PHAS-I by the mammalian target of rapamycin. *Science* 277: 99–101

32 Brunn GJ, Fadden P, Haystead TA, Lawrence JC Jr (1997) The mammalian Target of Rapamycin phosphorylates sites having a (Ser/Thr)-Pro motif and is activated by antibodies to a region near its COOH terminus. *J Biol Chem* 272: 32547–32550

33 Fadden P, Haystead TA, Lawrence JC Jr (1997) Identification of phosphorylation sites in the translational regulator, PHAS-I, that are controlled by insulin and rapamycin in rat adipocytes. *J Biol Chem* 272: 10240–10247

34 Gingras AC, Kennedy SG, O'Leary MA, Sonenberg N, Hay N (1998) 4E-BP1, a repressor of mRNA translation, is phosphorylated and inactivated by the Akt (PKB) signaling pathway. *Genes Dev* 12: 502–513

35 Scott PH, Brunn GJ, Kohn AD, Roth RA, Lawrence JC Jr (1998) Evidence of insulin-stimulated phosphorylation and activation of mammalian target of rapamycin by a protein kinase B signaling pathway. *Proc Natl Acad Sci USA* 95: 7772–7777

36 Brunn GJ, Williams J, Sabers C, Wiederrecht G, Lawrence JC Jr, Abraham RT (1996) Direct inhibition of the signaling functions of the mammalian target of rapamycin by the phosphoinositide 3-kinase inhibitors, wortmannin and LY294002. *EMBO J* 15: 5256–5267

37 Sarkaria JN, Tibbetts RS, Busby EC, Kennedy AP, Hill DE, Abraham RT (1998) Inhibition of phosphoinositide 3-kinase related kinases by the radiosensitizing agent wortmannin. *Cancer Res* 58: 4375–4382

Constitutive expression of a tumor suppressor leads to tumor regression in a xenograft model

Catherine Adams Burton[1], John Boylan[2], Candy Robinson[2], Janet Kerr[2] and Pamela Benfield[1]

[1]DuPont Pharmaceuticals Company, 500 S. Ridgeway Avenue, G-205 Glenolden, PA 19036, USA; [2]DuPont Pharmaceuticals Company, Research and Development Experimental Station, Wilmington, DE 19880-0440, USA

Introduction

The machinery of the cell cycle provides a mechanism for the duplication of cellular DNA during cell division and the appropriate distribution of this DNA to resulting daughter cells. It is important for cell survival that this process occurs in a highly regulated and controlled manner to ensure the accurate transmission of genetic material. Dividing eukaryotic cells are equipped with surveillance mechanisms to ensure that cell cycle progression does not occur if conditions are inappropriate, for example, if DNA is damaged or nucleotide supplies are limiting. These mechanisms have collectively been referred to as checkpoint control. Failure of checkpoint control leads to inappropriate cell division and the accumulation of DNA damage that is the hallmark of human tumor cells [4, 5].

The cell cycle is traditionally regarded as falling into four phases (Fig. 1). S phase represents the stage in the cycle when DNA replication occurs. This replicated DNA is segregated into two daughter cells during M phase, ending in final division of the cell at mitosis. Between these two phases are intervals originally regarded as "gaps", G_1 between mitosis and S phase, and G_2 between S phase and mitosis. Cell cycle progression is driven by the sequential activation of a family of kinases, the cyclin dependent kinases (CDKs). As their name implies this is a heterodimeric family of kinases which require an associated cyclin subunit for activity. Different cyclin/CDK pairs are responsible for driving progression through each phase of the cell cycle. Cyclin D in association with CDKs 4 and 6, together with cyclin E/CDK2, play a major role in driving cells through the G_1/S transition. Cyclins E and A along with CDK2 are important for S phase progression. Cyclins A and B along with CDK1 (also known as CDC2) drive cells through G_2 and on through mitosis (for reviews see [6, 7]).

The protein substrates for each of the cyclin/CDKs are still a subject of much research and are largely unidentified. However, a key substrate for the cyclin D/

Inflammatory Processes: Molecular Mechanisms and Therapeutic Opportunities, edited by L. Gordon Letts and Douglas W. Morgan
© 2000 Birkhäuser Verlag Basel/Switzerland

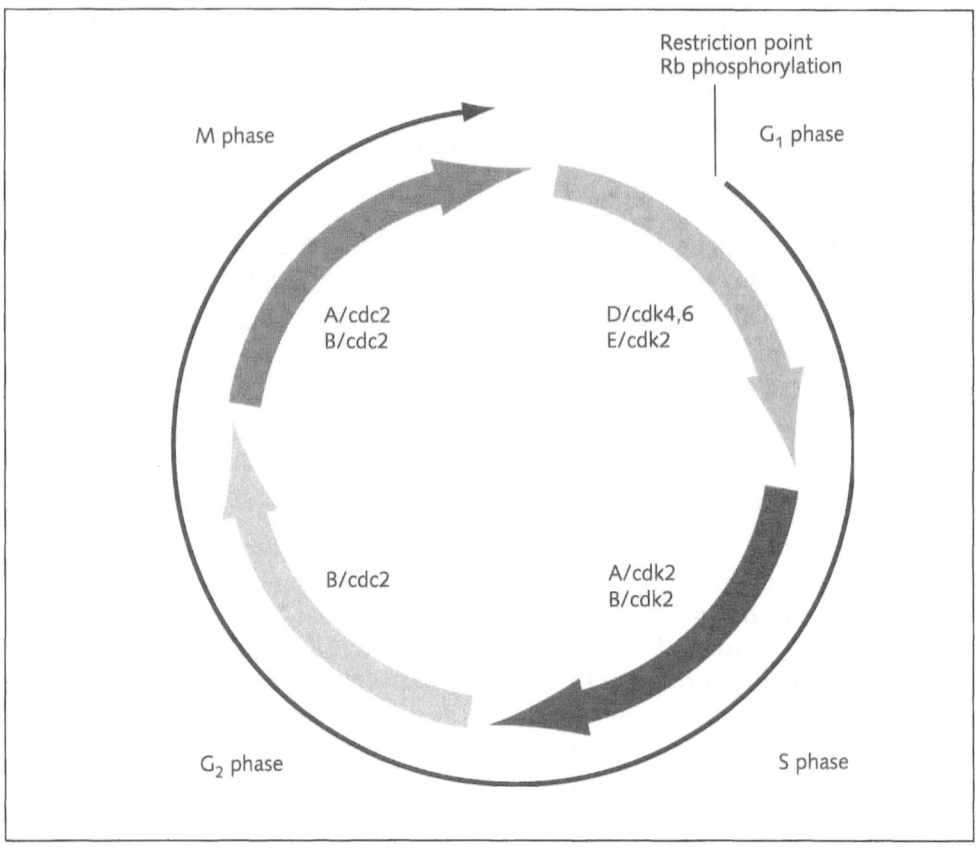

Figure 1
Schematic representation of the major phases of the eukaryotic cell cycle. Cyclin/CDK part-
ners responsible for driving cell cycle progression through each phase are shown in the cen-
ter of the circle. Times taken for an average cell to pass through each phase of the cycle are
not shown to scale.

CDK4,6 complexes is the tumor suppressor gene product, retinoblastoma (Rb) [8]. Phosphorylation of Rb occurs as cells pass through the G_1/S transition. Rb remains phosphorylated throughout the remainder of the cell cycle until it becomes dephosphorylated at mitosis. Phosphorylation of Rb corresponds to passage of cells through the restriction point. The restriction point represents a key decision point in cell cycle control. After passage through this point, cells become independent of growth factor stimulation for further cell cycle progression. One key feature of human tumor cells is that they have lost restriction point control and commit to uncontrolled cell cycle entry.

Activation of cyclin/CDK activity is subjected to several control mechanisms. CDK activity is subject to both positive and negative control by phosphorylation by upstream kinases. In addition, cells synthesize a family of small protein inhibitors of CDK activity which serve as natural regulators of cell cycle progression. These fall into two families: the p21/p27 gene family of regulators which have the ability to inhibit multiple cyclin/CDK pairs [9], and the p16 (MTS-1, INK4) gene family whose members are specific inhibitors of CDKs 4 and 6 [3, 10]. The MTS-1/INK4 gene has the ability, by alternate splicing, to engage two different reading frames and encode two different gene products [1, 2], the p16 inhibitor itself and a separate gene product, p19ARF [11, 12]. P19ARF acts to regulate p53 function [13], so that the MTS-1/INK4 locus has the unique ability to impact two tumor suppressor gene pathways of importance to human cancer, the Rb pathway and the p53 pathway [14]. Not surprisingly, the p16 locus is found mutated in a large percentage of human cancers [15–17], and loss of p16 locus function has been shown to be essential for the transforming activity of several other oncogenes, e.g. ras [18–20].

Given that loss of p16 function is a common event in human tumorigenesis, we asked what the impact of constitutive expression of p16 activity would be to human tumor cells grown both in monolayer culture and also grown as tumor xenografts in nude mice. These experiments are relevant to the potential for p16 mimics as therapies for human cancer.

Results and discussion

Human p16 was cloned into the mamalian expression vector (pcDNA3) and introduced by transient transfection into a series of human tumor cell lines. Empty vector was used as the control. Cell lines were chosen that were representative of different human cancers and for each cancer type two cell lines were tested that differed in their Rb status. The cell lines chosen were: breast carcinoma, MDA-MB-468 (Rb −ve), MDA-MB-453 (Rb +ve), osteosarcoma, SAOS-2 (Rb −ve), U2-OS (Rb +ve), leiomyosarcoma, SKUT-1A (Rb −ve), SKUT-1B (Rb +ve). Cell lines were obtained from the ATCC and propagated in the optimal medium suggested. 2×10^5 cells were plated and 24 h later transfected with 2 µg DNA using 10 µl lipofectamine in Optim-Mem. 2 h later an equal volume of growth medium was added containing 20% fetal calf serum. After 15 h incubation, cells were washed and growth medium replaced. 48 h later, cells from each transfection were trypsinized, counted and an equal number of cells were plated in triplicate in the presence of neomycin. Neomycin resistant colonies were scored seven days later. In Figure 2 results are expressed as the percent reduction in colony formation relative to the vector control. Efficient inhibition of colony formation was seen in each of the Rb positive cell lines, with no inhibition occurring in the "paired" Rb negative cell line. This result is in agreement with that reported by others [21–24] and is consistent

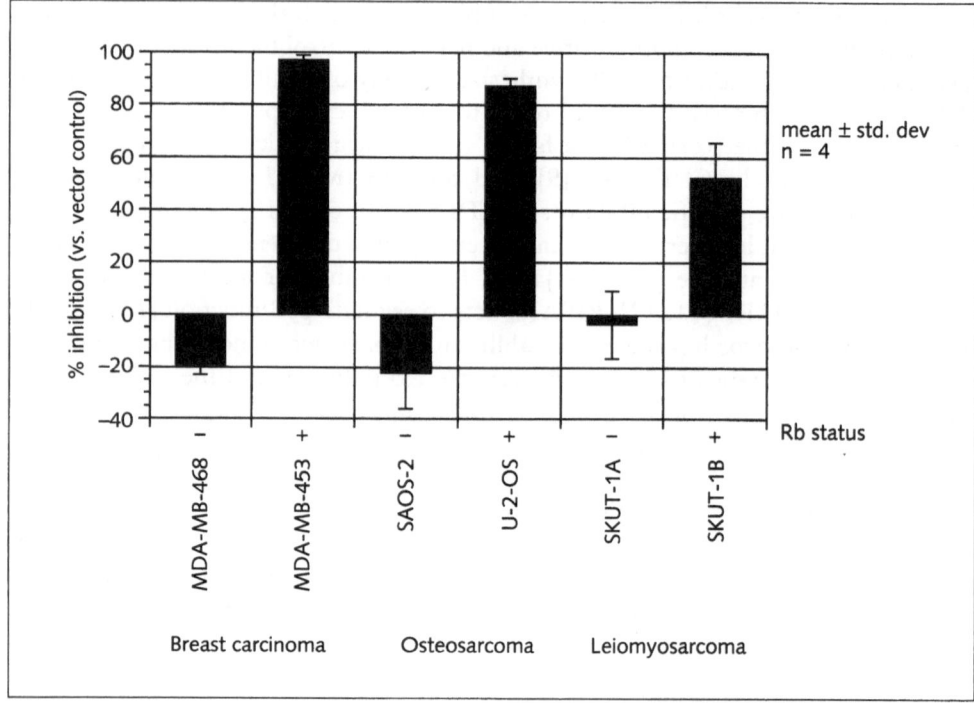

Figure 2
Effect of p16 transfection in Rb ± cell line pairs. The bar graphs show the percent inhibition of colony formation in each individual cell line in the presence of exogenously expressed p16. The cell lines used in the experiment and the Rb status of these cell lines is indicated at the bottom of the figure.

with the role of p16 as a specific inhibitor of CDK4/6, and Rb as the principal substrate for CDK4/6 cyclin complexes. Cells lacking Rb have become independent of CDK4/6 for cell cycle progression and therefore, insensitive to the impact of p16.

The above experiment shows that p16 expression can result in inhibition of colony formation and that this inhibition is Rb dependent. However, it does not address the outcome of p16 induction in non-colony forming cells, i.e. does p16 induction lead to cell cycle inhibition or cell death? To address this issue, p16 was cloned into a vector that would allow reversible induction of p16 in a controlled manner. The vector (p10.3hgh) was chosen whereby p16 could be repressed in the presence of tetracycline and induced upon tetracycline withdrawal [25]. A series of stable cell lines was created using this vector in the H358 tumor cell background. H358 cells are derived from a human non-small cell lung carcinoma. They are p53 deficient and wild type for Rb. They contain mutant ras and can form tumors in

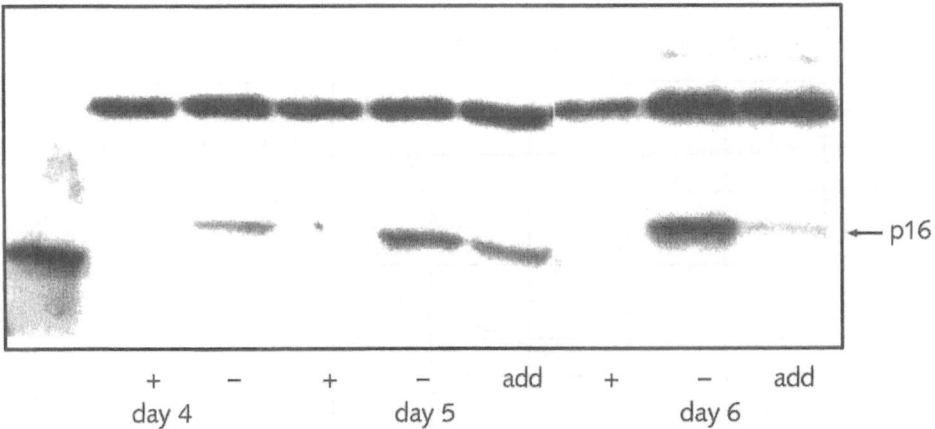

Figure 3
Western analysis of p16 expression in the H358p16#26 cell line. Cells were grown in the presence and absence of tetracycline for the number of days indicated at the bottom of the figure. The migration position of p16 is indicated by the arrow on the right. The first lane of the figure corresponds to analysis of recombinant p16 protein with an N-terminal deletion as described in the text and serves as a positive control for antibody recognition.

nude mice [26]. Figure 3 shows the result of analysis of one cell line from this series, clone #26. This figure shows a Western blot analysis of whole cell extracts of the H358p16#26 cell line grown in the presence and absence of 10 ng/ml tetracycline. The blot is probed with anti-p16 antibody. The running position of p16 is indicated by the arrow at the right of the figure. Samples were normalized for cell number and a non-specific band that cross hybridizes with the antibody and that runs above the p16, serves as an internal control for protein loading. The band in the lane at the far left of the figure is derived from p16 control protein produced *in vitro* using a p16 expression plasmid that drives the expression of p16 with a small N-terminal truncation. This control protein serves as a positive control for the anti-p16 antibody. In the presence of 10 ng/ml tetracycline, p16 expression in H358p16#26 cells is undetectable. Upon withdrawal of tetracycline, p16 expression can clearly be detected by day 4 of antibiotic removal. Expression continues to increase on days 5 and 6. Re-addition of tetracycline to the cell culture on day 4 results in repression of p16 expression by day 5 and almost total loss of expression by day 6. This experiment indicates that p16 expression can be controlled reversibly in response to tetracycline in this H358p16#26 cell line.

The impact of p16 expression on H358 cell growth in clone 26 is shown in Figure 4. This graph shows the impact of p16 expression on cell number as a function

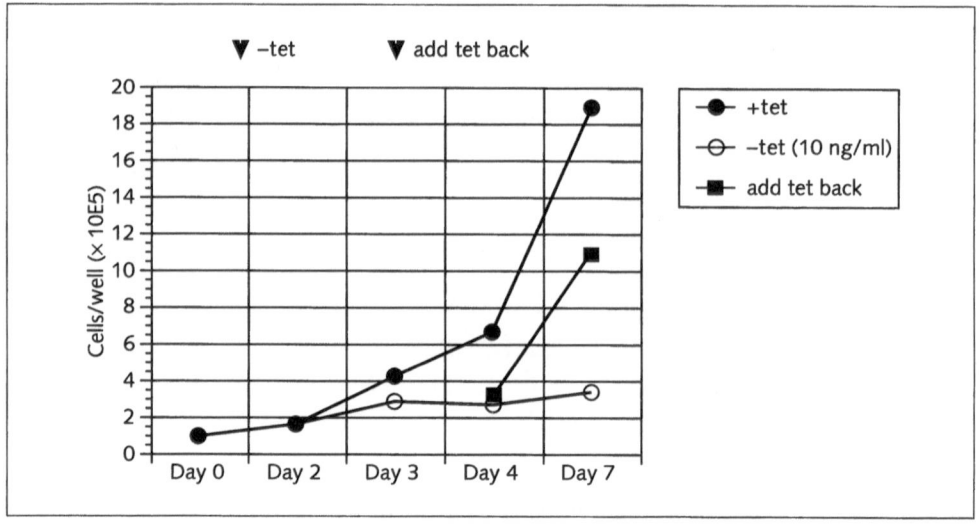

Figure 4

Growth curves for the H358p16#26 cell line grown in the presence and absence of tetracy-cline as indicated at the right of the figure. In the tet add back experiment, cells were grown in the absence of tetracycline until day3 as indicated and then tetracycline (10 ng/ml) was readded to the medium to resuppress p16 expression.

of time. Clone 26 cells grown in the presence of 10 ng/ml tetracycline, where p16 expression is repressed, show an exponential increase in cell number. In the absence of tetracycline, p16 is induced and cell growth is almost totally repressed. Under these conditions cells appear morphologically changed. They take on a "flat cell phenotype" typical of senescent cells. FACS analysis indicates that these cells are arrested in G_1 (data not shown). Consistent with these cells being in a reversibly arrested state, if tetracycline is added back on day 3, p16 is repressed and cell number increases once more.

P16 mimics represent a potentially important approach to cancer therapy since they should restore aspects of G_1 checkpoint control lacking in cancer cells. However, the question remained as to whether such mimics would be tumor static, or whether they may support tumor regression. Given that p16 induction in the H358 cell line appeared to result in reversible G_1 arrest, we asked what the impact of this arrest might be in a tumor-like setting. The H358p16#26 cell line was propagated as tumors in nude mice. 2×10^6 cells were injected subcutaneously into the flank of Swiss female nude mice and tumors allowed to form. Each experimental group contained five animals. Tumor burden was estimated by caliper measurements and these measurements were used to calculate tumor weights using standard methods [27]. Animals bearing tumors that represented > 10% of their body weight were terminated.

	Group 1	Group 2	Group 3	Group 4
	Tumor mass (mm³) mean ± SEM			
Day 0		**Cells injected S.C.***		
Day 20	14 ± 2.5	60 ± 12	66 ± 12	43 ± 11.4
Day 40	too small	8.4 ± 0.4	7.2 ± 1.3	87 ± 76
Day 51	one tumor	15.2 ± 7.2	45.2 ± 13	105.5 ± 13.1

*2 × 10⁶ two places on flank ☐ −tet, p16 induced

21 Day 0.7 µg/day release pellets ☐ +tet, p16 repressed

Figure 5
Effect of p16 induction on H358p16#26 grown in xenografts. The experiment was performed as described in the text. Mean calculated tumor mass (mm³) at each time point for each experimental group is shown in the table. Periods of time when tetracycline is withdrawn (p16 is induced) are indicated by hatched filling in the table.

In this experiment (Fig. 5) group 4 animals were maintained on 21 day release tetracycline pellets that would deliver 0.7 µg tetracycline per day. Under these conditions p16 expression in the tumor cells should be repressed. As anticipated group 4 animals showed continued tumor growth during the 51 day time-course of the experiment. By contrast, group 1 animals received no tetracycline pellets. In these animals p16 induction should be maintained throughout the experiment. In these animals no sustained tumor growth was observed. Small tumors were evaluated on day 20, but were too small to measure on days 40 and 51.

Two additional groups of animals were generated to test further the impact of p16 expression on tumor growth and survival in the xenograft setting. For the first 21 days, group 2 animals were maintained in the presence of tetracycline to repress p16 expression. During this period, tumor growth was observed, and tumors attained a size similar to that seen in group 4 control animals. On day 21, the tetra-cycline pellet was not refreshed so that thereafter tetracycline levels fell, and p16 expression was induced. In these animals a regression in tumor size was observed on day 40 relative to the day 21 value, and this regression was maintained out to day 51. Group 3 animals were treated similarly to group 2 animals until day 40 and showed a similar pattern of tumor growth to day 20, followed by regression on day 40. At this time, a new tetracylcine pellet was implanted in the animals in this group to repress p16 induction and determine if regression was reversible. In these animals, renewed tumor growth was seen by day 51, suggesting that maintenance of tumor regression required the continued expression of p16, at least over this time period.

Collectively these results indicate that in the H358 cell line p16 induction leads to a reversible G_1 arrest in cells in culture, and that this arrest translates to a tumor regression rather than tumor stasis in the xenograft setting. We are currently assessing the mechanism of this regression. Possibly, in the different environment presented in the xenograft, p16 induction in H358 cells leads to tumor cell apoptosis rather than arrest. Regrowth of tumors upon p16 repression would then result from incomplete apoptosis in the time frame of this experiment. It would be interesting to determine if more sustained p16 expression eventually results in an irreversible tumor regression. Alternatively host mechanisms may contribute to tumor clearance in the arrested state. Finally, in these experiments p16 expression is limited to the tumor tissue and experiments need to be designed to address the likely toxic impact of more global expression of a p16 mimetic in the context of a tumor bearing animal, and the likelihood of achieving a practical therapeutic index.

Nevertheless these experiments are among the first to examine the impact of correction of a tumor suppressor defect in the context of a tumor bearing animal. They strongly support the conclusion that p16 mimics may drive tumor regressions and not simply tumor stasis. Furthermore, given that the cell line used in these experiments is p53 deficient they suggest that these regressions should be possible independent of tumor p53 status. These results in turn support the notion that mimics of p16 may have a desirable profile as cancer therapeutics.

References

1   Kamb A, Gruis NA, Weaver-Feldhaus J, Liu Q, Harshman K, Tavtigian SV, Stockert E, Day RS 3rd, Johnson BE, Skolnick MH (1994) A cell cycle regulator potentially involved in the genesis of many tumor types. *Science* 264: 344–345

2   Larsen CJ (1997) Contribution of the dual coding capacity of the p16INK4a/MTS1/CDKN2 locus to human malignancies. *Prog Cell Cycle Res* 3: 109–124

3   Serrano M, Hannon GJ, Beach D (1993) A new regulatory motif in cell-cycle control causing specific inhibition of cyclin D/CDK4. *Nature* 366: 704–707

4   Hartwell LH, Kastan MB (1994) Cell cycle control and cancer. *Science* 266: 1821–1828

5   Hartwell L (1992) Defects in a cell cycle checkpoint may be responsible for the genomic instability of cancer cells. *Cell* 71: 543–546

6   Murray AW (1994) Cyclin dependent kinases: regulators of the cell cycle and more. *Current Biology* 1: 191–195

7   Pines J (1995) Cyclins and cyclin-dependent kinases: Theme and variations. *Adv in Cancer Res* 66: 181–212

8   Lukas J, Bartkova J, Rohde M, Strauss M, Bartek J (1995) Cyclin D1 is dispensible for G1 control in retinoblastoma gene-deficient cells independently of cdk4 activity. *Mol Cell Biol* 15: 2600–2611

9   Sherr CJ, Roberts JM (1995) Inhibitors of mammalian G1 cyclin-dependent kinases. *Genes Dev* 9: 1149–1163

10   Serrano M (1997) The tumor suppressor protein p16INK4a. *Exp Cell Res* 7–13

11   Quelle DE, Zindy F, Ashmun RA, Sherr CJ (1995) Alternative reading frames of the INK4a tumor suppressor gene encode two unrelated proteins capable of inducing cell cycle arrest. *Cell* 83: 993–1000

12   Chin L, Pomerantz J, DePinho RA (1998) The INK4a/ARF tumor suppressor gene – two products – two pathways. *Trends Biochem Sci* 23: 291–296

13   Pomerantz J, Schreiber-Agus N, Liegeois NJ, Silverman A, Alland L, Chin L, Potes J, Chen K, Orlow I, Lee HW, Cordon-Cardo C, DePinho RA (1998) The Ink4a tumor suppressor gene product, p19Arf, interacts with MDM2 and neutralizes MDM2's inhibition of p53. *Cell* 92: 713–723

14   Zhang Y, Xiong Y, Yarbrough WG (1998) ARF promotes MDM2 degradation and stabilizes p53: ARF-INK4a locus deletion impairs both the Rb and p53 tumor suppression pathways. *Cell* 92: 725–734

15   Gazzeri S, Della Valle V, Chaussade L, Brambilla C, Larsen CJ, Brambilla E (1998) The human p19ARF protein encoded by the beta transcript of the p16INK4a gene is frequently lost in small cell lung cancer. *Cancer Res* 58: 3926–3931

16   Vonlanthen S, Heighway J, Tschan MP, Borner MM, Altermatt HJ, Kappeler A, Tobler A, Fey MF, Thatcher N, Yarbrough WG, Betticher DC (1998) Expression of p16INK4a/p16α and p19ARF/p16β is frequently altered in non-small cell lung cancer and correlates with p53 overexpression. *Oncogene* 17: 2779–2785

17   Gorgoulis VG, Zacharatos P, Kotsinas A, Liloglou T, Kyroudi A, Veslemes M, Rassidakis A, Halazonitis TD, Field JK, Kittas C (1998) Alterations of the p16-pRb pathway and the chromosome locus 9p21-22 in non-small-cell lung carcinomas: Relationship with p53 and MDM2 protein expression. *Am J Pathol* 153: 1749–1765

18   Serrano M, Gomez-Lahoz E, DePinho RA, Beach D, Bar-Sagi D (1995) Inhibition of ras-induced proliferation and cellular transformation by p16INK4. *Science* 267: 249–252

19   Serrano M, Lin AW, McCurrach ME, Beach D, Lowe SW (1997) Oncogenic ras promotes premature cell senescence associated with accumulation of p53 and p16INK4a. *Cell* 88: 593–602

20 Haas K, Staller P, Geisen C, Bartek J, Eilers M, Moroy T (1997) Mutual requirement of CDK4 and Myc in malignant transformation: evidence for cyclin D1/CDK4 and P16INK4a as upstream regulators of Myc. *Oncogene* 15: 179–192

21 Medema RH, Herrara RE, Lam P, Weinberg RA (1995) Growth suppression by p16ink4 requires functional retinoblastoma protein. *Proc Natl Acad Sci USA* 92: 6289–6293

22 Jin X, Nguyen D, Zhang WW, Kyritsis AP, Roth JA (1995) Cell cycle arrest and inhibition of tumor cell proliferation by the p16INK4 gene mediated by an adenovirus vector. *Cancer Res* 55: 3250–3253

23 Spillare EA, Okamoto A, Hagiwara K, Demetrick DJ, Serrano M, Beach D, Harris CC (1996) Suppression of growth *in vitro* and tumorigenicity *in vivo* of human carcinoma cell lines by transfected p16INK4. *Mol Carcinog* 16: 53–60

24 Craig C, Kim M, Ohri E, Wersto R, Katayose D, Li Z, Choi YH, Mudahar B, Srivastava S, Seth P, Cowan K (1997) Effects of the adenovirus-mediated p16INK4A expression on cell cycle arrest are determined by endogenous p16 and Rb status in human cancer cells. *Oncogene* 16: 265–272

25 Gossen M, Bujard H (1992) Tight control of gene expression in mammalian cells by tetracycline responsive promoters. *Proc Natl Acad Sci USA* 89: 5547–5551

26 Alemany R, Ruan S, Kataoka M, Koch PE, Mukhopadhyay T, Cristiano RJ, Roth JA, Zhang WW (1996) Growth inhibitory effect of anti-K-ras adenovirus on lung cancer cells. *Cancer Gene Ther* 3: 296–301

27 Dykes DJ, Abbott BJ, Mayo JG, Harrison Jr SD, Laster Jr WR, Simpson-Herren L, Griswold Jr DP (1992) Development of human tumor xenograft models for *in vivo* evaluation of new antitumor drugs. *Contrib Oncol* 42: 1–22

Macrophage metalloproteinases in destructive inflammatory diseases

Steven D. Shapiro

Departments of Pediatrics, Medicine, and Cell Biology and Physiology, Washington University School of Medicine at Barnes-Jewish Hospital, St. Louis, MO 63110, USA

Introduction

Expression of matrix metalloproteinases (MMPs) is associated with a variety of destructive diseases including atherosclerotic plaque rupture, abdominal aortic aneurysms, tumor invasion, arthritis, and emphysema. This has led to the hypothesis that aberrant expression of MMPs causes tissue destruction. The macrophage, intimately associated with these inflammatory diseases is a rich source of MMPs. Interestingly, both emphysema and aortic aneurysms are associated with macrophage infiltration and elastic fiber destruction. This paper will review the potential roles of macrophage MMPs in general, and macrophage elastase (MMP-12) in particular, in the development of aneurysm formation and emphysema. The role of gene targeting will be discussed as a method to perform controlled experiments in mammals to determine the effects of macrophage MMPs in these disease processes.

Macrophage matrix metalloproteinases

Matrix metalloproteinases represent a family of matrix degrading enzymes with structural similarities. They require coordination of a zinc ion at the active site for catalysis, and their activity is specifically inhibited by the tissue inhibitors of matrix metalloproteinases (TIMPs 1–4). Of the roughly 20 MMPs described, macrophages have the capacity to produce several MMPs, including collagenase-1 (MMP-1), stromelysin-1 (MMP-3), matrilysin (MMP-7), gelatinase B (MMP-9), macrophage elastase (MMP-12), and MT1-MMP (MMP-14). Mice have a similar profile of MMPs except that macrophage elastase appears to be the predominant mouse macrophage MMP.

Inflammatory Processes: Molecular Mechanisms and Therapeutic Opportunities, edited by L. Gordon Letts and Douglas W. Morgan

Macrophage elastase (MMP-12)

MMP-12 was first detected in 1975 when Werb and Gordon identified elastolytic activity in mouse peritoneal macrophage conditioned media [1]. Subsequently, in 1981, Banda and Werb purified a 22 kDa metal-dependent proteinase that was responsible for this activity [2]. Cloning of the murine cDNA (MME) from a murine macrophage (P388D1) library demonstrated that macrophage elastase was a distinct member of the MMP family with 33–49% amino acid homology with other matrix metalloproteinases [3]. The human orthologue of macrophage elastase (HME) was then cloned from a cDNA library derived from human alveolar macrophages of a cigarette smoker [4]. The cDNAs for human and murine macrophage elastase have 74% homology; there is 64% identity between the enzymes at the amino acid level.

MMP-12 shares many features typical of MMPs including its domain structure, chromosomal location within the MMP gene cluster on human chromosome 11q22, and its capacity to potently hydrolyze a broad spectrum of extracellular matrix components (Leu preference in the P1' position) excluding interstitial collagens [5]. MMP-12 is also unique with respect to its predominantly macrophage-specific pattern of expression and the ability to readily shed its C-terminal domain upon processing.

Macrophages of MMP-12$^{-/-}$ mice have a markedly diminished capacity to degrade extracellular matrix components [5]. MMP-12$^{-/-}$ macrophages are essentially unable to penetrate reconstituted basement membranes both *in vitro* and *in vivo*. The prominent expression of MMP-12 in mouse macrophages has made MMP-12$^{-/-}$ mice an excellent model system for determining the role of extracellular macrophage-mediated proteolysis in a variety of (patho)biological processes.

Vascular aneurysms

Abdominal aortic aneurysms (AAA) affect 2–9% of adults greater than 65 years of age. AAAs are associated with aging, atherosclerosis, cigarette smoking, and male gender. AAAs are believed to result from structural remodeling of the elastin-rich aortic wall in association with chronic transmural inflammation. Mononuclear cell infiltration in the aortic media associated with elastic fiber destruction might be of particular importance. MMP-9 [6] and macrophage elastase [7] were found to be prominently expressed in macrophages associated with elastic fiber disruption in specimens of human abdominal aortic aneurysm. Production of macrophage elastase was increased seven-fold in patients with aneurysms, and expression was localized to the active "transition zone" in the media. This is the region adjacent to normal aorta where there is active remodeling and elastin degradation. Unlike other

MMPs, macrophage elastase also specifically bound to fragmented, but not intact, elastic fibers in this zone. *In vitro* studies, confirmed that macrophage elastase has a greater binding affinity for elastin than other elastases. These findings suggest that macrophage elastase might play a central role in aneurysm formation in humans.

Mice with a targeted disruption of apolipoprotein E gene (ApoE$^{-/-}$) have a delayed clearance of lipoproteins, and when fed a Western diet develop serum cholesterol levels of 1,400–2,000 mg/dl, and develop fatty streaks progressing to fibrous plaques at branch points of major vessels. This is associated with macrophage recruitment causing disruption of the medial external elastic lamina (EEL) and aortic microaneurysm formation.

To investigate the role of plasminogen activators [(PA), tissue-type PA (t-PA) and urokinase-type (u-PA)] in aneurysms and atherosclerosis, Carmeleit and colleagues crossed ApoE$^{-/-}$ mice with u-PA$^{-/-}$ and t-PA$^{-/-}$ mice. ApoE$^{-/-}$ X u-PA$^{-/-}$ mice (but not ApoE$^{-/-}$ or ApoE$^{-/-}$X t-PA$^{-/-}$) were protected from macrophage-mediated destruction of medial external elastic lamina (EEL) and microaneurysm formation [8]. It appears that local production of plasmin (by u-PA) is required to activate pro-MME and perhaps other MMPs. In the absence of plasmin, macrophages line-up but do not penetrate or disrupt the EEL. This is consistent with earlier findings that macrophages of MME$^{-/-}$ mice cannot penetrate basement membranes or degrade [9]. These results suggest that plasmin is required for MMP activation in this model, and that MMPs, particularly MME, are responsible for matrix destruction and macrophage infiltration associated with atherosclerotic microaneurysm formation and potentially plaque rupture.

Pulmonary emphysema

Pulmonary emphysema is a major component of the morbidity and mortality of chronic obstructive pulmonary disease (COPD), a condition that afflicts more than 14 million persons in the US and has become the fourth leading cause of death. The vast majority of patients with COPD are cigarette smokers, but only ~ 15% of cigarette smokers present to physicians with COPD, suggesting that additional genetic and environmental factors contribute to this disease process. Given the large increase in smoking in many foreign countries, COPD will become a larger worldwide problem in the ensuing years [10].

Emphysema is defined as enlargement of peripheral airspaces of the lung including respiratory bronchioles, alveolar ducts, and alveoli, accompanied by destruction of the walls of these structures. Inherited deficiency of α_1-antitrypsin, the primary inhibitor of neutrophil elastase, predisposes individuals to early onset emphysema, and intrapulmonary instillation of elastolytic enzymes in experimental animals causes emphysema. Together, these findings led to the elastase:antielastase hypothesis for the pathogenesis of emphysema which has been the prevailing hypothesis for over

30 years. However, macrophages, not neutrophils, are the most abundant defense cell in the lung both under normal conditions and in the lungs of smokers. The capacity of macrophages to degrade elastin, and to hence contribute to emphysema, was controversial until Chapman and colleagues [11] identified elastolytic cysteine proteinases. Subsequently, we found elastolytic MMPs produced by alveolar macrophages [12]. In our studies the macrophage elastolytic activity was inhibited by the TIMPs, therefore we focused on the role of MMPs, particularly macrophage elastase, in the pathogenesis of emphysema.

Macrophage elastase, nearly undetectable in normal macrophages, is expressed in human alveolar macrophages of cigarette smokers. We also detect HME by immunohistochemistry and in situ hybridization in macrophages in patients with emphysema, but not normal lung tissue. To determine directly the contribution of macrophage elastase to emphysema we (1) developed a murine model of cigarette smoke-induced emphysema, (2) generated macrophage elastase-deficient (MME$^{-/-}$) mice by gene-targeting, and (3) subjected MME$^{-/-}$ mice and wild-type (MME$^{+/+}$) littermates to chronic cigarette smoke exposure [13]. We found that in contrast to MMP-12$^{+/+}$ mice, mice lacking macrophage elastase (MMP-12$^{-/-}$) did not develop emphysema. Surprisingly, MMP-12$^{-/-}$ mice also failed to recruit macrophages into their lungs in response to cigarette smoke. Monthly intratracheal instillation of monocyte chemoattractant protein-1 to smoke exposed MMP-12$^{-/-}$ mice resulted in recruitment of MMP-12$^{-/-}$ alveolar macrophages but failed to cause airspace enlargement. Thus, macrophage elastase is required for both macrophage accumulation and emphysema resulting from chronic inhalation of cigarette smoke. Our current working model is that cigarette smoke induces constitutive macrophages to produce MME which cleaves elastin generating fragments chemotactic for monocytes. This positive feedback loop perpetuates macrophage accumulation and lung destruction.

References

1   Werb Z, Gordon S (1975) Elastase secretion by stimulated macrophages. *J Exp Med* 142: 361–377

2   Banda MJ, Werb Z (1981) Mouse macrophage elastase. Purification and characterization as a metalloproteinase. *Biochem J* 193: 589–605

3   Shapiro SD, Griffin G, Gilbert DJ, Jenkins NA, Copeland NG, Welgus HG, Senior RM, Ley TJ (1992) Molecular cloning, chromosomal localization and bacterial expression of a novel murine macrophage metalloelastase. *J Biol Chem* 267: 4664–4671

4   Shapiro SD, Kobayashi D, Ley T (1993) Cloning and characterization of a unique elastolytic metalloproteinase produced by human alveolar macrophages. *J Biol Chem* 268: 23824–23829

5   Gronski TJ, Martin R, Kobayashi DK, Walsh BC, Holman MC, Van Wart HE, Shapiro

SD (1997) Hydrolysis of a broad spectrum of extracellular matrix proteins by human macrophage elastase. *J Biol Chem* 272: 12189–12194

6   Thompson RW, Mertens RA, Liao S, Holmes DR, Mecham RP, Welgus HG, Parks WC (1995) Production and localization of 92-kD gelatinase in abdominal aortic aneurysms: an elastolytic metalloproteinase expressed by aneurysm-infiltrating macrophages. *J Clin Invest* 96: 318–326

7   Curci JA, Liao S, Huffman MD, Shapiro SD, Thompson RW (1998) Elevated production of macrophage elastase (MMP-12) in abdominal aortic aneurysms and its specific localization to elastic fiber fragments within the degenerating aortic media. *J Clin Invest; in press*

8   Carmeleit P, Moons L, Lijnen R, Crawley J, Tipping P, Drew A, Eeckhout Y, Shapiro SD, Lupu F, Collen D (1997) Plasmin predisposes to atherosclerotic aneurysm formation by activation of matrix metalloproteinases. *Nature Genetics* 17: 439–444

9   Shipley JM, Wesselschmidt RL, Kobayashi DK, Ley TJ, Shapiro SD (1996) Metalloelastase is required for macrophage-mediated proteolysis and matrix invasion in mice. *Proc Natl Acad Sci* 93: 3942–3946

10   Bartecchi C, MacKenzie T, Schrier R (1994) The human costs of tobacco use. *N Engl J Med* 330: 907–912 and 975–980

11   Chapman HAJ, Stone OL (1984) Comparison of live human neutrophil and alveolar macrophage elastolytic activity *in vitro*. Relative resistance of macrophage elastolytic activity to serum and alveolar proteinase inhibitors. *J Clin Invest* 74: 1693–1700

12   Senior RM, Griffin GL, Fliszar CJ, Shapiro SD, Goldberg GI, Welgus HG (1991) Human 92-kilodalton and 72-kilodalton type IV collagenases are elastases. *J Biol Chem* 266: 7870–7875

13   Hautamaki RD, Kobayashi DK, Senior RM, Shapiro SD (1997) Macrophage elastase is required for cigarette smoke-induced emphysema in mice. *Science* 277: 2002–2004

Lymphotoxin in inflammation and lymphoid organ development: Variations on a theme

Nancy H. Ruddle

Yale University School of Medicine, Department of Epidemiology and Public Health and Immunobiology, 815 LEPH, New Haven, CT 06520-8034, USA

Introduction

Members of the LT/TNF family have long been implicated in inflammation through experimental studies of autoimmune diseases and transgenic mice (reviewed in [1]). In the case of autoimmune inflammation, the lesion is initiated by antigen-specific T cells which recruit additional T cells, B cells, and macrophages. The consequences of inflammation include tissue damage and in many autoimmune diseases the inflammation becomes chronic, eventually developing into "tertiary lymphoid organs", with the infiltrates taking on the appearance of new lymphoid organs, a phenomenon we have termed: lymphoid neogenesis [2]. It is possible that these newly formed local lymphoid organs contribute to clinical relapses and epitope spreading which occurs in the course of many autoimmune diseases. In these situations the individual reacts not only to the immunizing auto-antigen, but also over time to additional determinants within that antigen and to unrelated molecules that also comprise the target organ [3]. We suggest that this phenomenon occurs within the local target organ in the course of an inflammatory reaction within the newly organized lymphoid tissue and that cytokines contribute to this phenomenon *via* mechanisms similar to those they employ in lymphoid organ development.

The LT/TNF family

There are three members of the immediate LT/TNF family comprising a complex that maps within the major histocompatibility complex (MHC) in man (chromosome 6) and mouse (chromosome 17). TNFα, produced as a Type II membrane-bound protein, that is clipped and released by a TNFα converting enzyme (TACE), is a product of macrophages and also T cells. LT is secreted as a homotrimer and, like TNFα, binds to TNF receptor (TNFR) I and II, resulting in its functional simi-

Inflammatory Processes: Molecular Mechanisms and Therapeutic Opportunities, edited by L. Gordon Letts and Douglas W. Morgan
© 2000 Birkhäuser Verlag Basel/Switzerland

larity to TNFα. However, it also forms a heterotrimer with LTβ, a Type II transmembrane protein, allowing it to bind to the LTβR. The members of this family have been implicated in inflammation and also in the development of lymphoid organs. One of our goals is to understand the mechanisms of these process. LTα3 and TNFα3 induce adhesion molecules *in vitro* on a murine endothelial cell line, bEnd.3 [4]. These adhesion molecules include ICAM, VCAM, E-selectin, and MAdCAM, the mucosal addressin cellular adhesion molecule, a marker of all developing lymph nodes (LN) and mature mucosal LN and Peyer's patches (PP). LTα3 does not induce PNAd (peripheral node addressin), a marker of peripheral LN. LTα3 also induces chemokines including RANTES, IP-10, and MCP-1 from this cell line [4]. The expression of LTα as a transgene also results in induction of adhesion molecules typically thought of as involved in inflammation, such as VCAM and ICAM, but also those associated with lymphoid organs, namely MAdCAM and PNAd [2].

The role of the LT/TNF family in lymphoid organ development

As noted above, members of the LT/TNF family play crucial roles in lymphoid organ development (summarized in [5]). These activities are varied and involve combinatorial association of the ligands and their receptors. Most of the cytokines and their receptors are involved in splenic development. LTα1β2 through the LTβR is important for peripheral LN, whereas LTα3 is implicated more strongly in mucosal LN, such as the mesenteric and cervical LN. Neither the mechanism of these processes, nor the identity of the cells that make these cytokines is known in development.

The role of LT in EAE

Experimental autoimmune encephalomyelitis (EAE) is a murine model of multiple sclerosis that results after immunization of mice with components of spinal cord. Numerous lines of evidence implicate the LT/TNF family in this autoimmune disease. These include the necessity for production of LTα by T-cell clones that transfer EAE, inhibition of transfer of EAE by agents that inhibit LT and TNF or the LT/TNF receptors (TNFRI) [6–10], and the fact that mice deficient in LTα, but not LTβ, are resistant to EAE induced by myelin oligodendrocyte glycoprotein peptide 35-55 [11]. There has been some controversy concerning the roles of the individual family members regarding this disease when the various knock-out mice were studied and this could be in part a function of the various background strains and modes of immunization employed by the various authors (reviewed in [12]).

There are several avenues through which LT could contribute to EAE. These include: killing oligodendrocytes, providing help for antibody production, inducing inflammation through induction of adhesion molecules and chemokines, and providing a structure for antigen presentation within the central nervous system (CNS) and thus facilitating determinant spreading. The ability of LT to induce apoptosis in many different cell types including oligodendrocytes has been well documented [13] and will not be further addressed here. Instead, the emphasis will be on LT's activities that are apparent in development and inflammation. The first issue to be addressed is the necessity of LT for antibody production. Members of the LT/TNF family are crucial for germinal center formation and $LT\alpha^{-/-}$ and $LT\beta^{-/-}$ mice have lower titers of certain isotypes [14]. Thus, if antibodies to MOG are crucial for EAE and $LT\alpha^{-/-}$ mice have lower titers of such antibodies, then the defect in $LT\alpha^{-/-}$ mice with regard to EAE could be explained as a problem in humoral immunity. This point was addressed by evaluating the importance of antibody production in MOG induced EAE by studying mice that were deficient in antibody by their absence of surface IgM (μMT mice) [15]. Wild type (WT) mice and μMT mice were immunized with MOG peptide 35-55 in complete Freund's adjuvant (CFA) and injected with pertussis toxin twice and then boosted again with MOG in CFA. Mice in both groups of mice developed EAE of comparable maximum disease severity (2.8 vs 3.2), average day of onset (12.8 vs 11.3), and duration. Histologic examination of the CNS also revealed patterns and intensity of inflammation and demyelination that were indistinguishable [15]. These data, which are similar to those reported by others [16], indicate that antibody production is not crucial for MOG-induced EAE and suggest that any reduction in anti-MOG antibody production exhibited by the $LT\alpha^{-/-}$ mice is not an important contributing factor to their profound resistance to EAE.

It is likely that LT contributes importantly to EAE through its ability to induce inflammation. Accordingly, whereas the WT mice with MOG-induced EAE have extensive CNS inflammation with T cells, B cells, and macrophages, $LT\alpha^{-/-}$ mice have almost no inflammation and demyelination [11]. This is probably due to the fact that the normal induction of adhesion molecules [2, 4, 17] and chemokines [4] by $LT\alpha$ does not occur, and thus the inflammatory process is not set into motion.

Chronic autoimmune infiltrates have the characteristics of organized lymphoid tissue

It has been noted repeatedly that chronic autoimmune infiltrates take on the characteristics of organized lymphoid tissue. It is possible that these "new" lymphoid organs contribute to antigen presentation at the local site, and that cytokines, especially $LT\alpha$ with its crucial role in inflammation and lymphoid organ development, are the unifying mechanistic features of these processes. There are several instances in which autoimmune infiltrates take on the characteristics of "tertiary lymphoid organs". These include: myasthenia gravis, in which the thymus develops germinal centers, rheumatoid arthritis in which the joints contain T and B cells, multiple sclerosis and EAE in which the presence of blood vessels with the characteristics of high endothelial venules are seen, and the non obese diabetic mouse in which blood vessels with the antigenic characteristics of those seen in LN are apparent by their expression of MAdCAM-1 and PNAd (reviewed in [2]). It has also been noted in a LT-induced model of inflammation in which LTα is driven as a transgene by the rat insulin promoter (RIPLT mice) and is expressed in the kidney and pancreas resulting in infiltrates in those organs [18], that the infiltrates take on the functional and morphologic characteristics of lymphoid organs [2]. These features include segregation into B- and T-cell areas, the appearance of germinal centers especially after immunization, blood vessels with the morphologic and antigenic (MAdCAM and PNAd) characteristics of HEV, and the ability of cells in the infiltrates to respond with antibody production and immunoglobulin class switching after immunization with sheep red blood cells (SRBC) [2]. The commonality of these infiltrates and lymphoid organs is further emphasized in that the LT produced by these transgenic mice restores most LN to LTα$^{-/-}$ mice [19]. The as yet unanswered question is whether LT production in the CNS in the process of EAE results in lymphoid accumulations with the characteristics of lymphoid organs, and whether these new lymphoid organs present auto-antigens at the local site, contributing to the phenomenon of determinant spreading.

In conclusion, LT/TNF family members contribute to inflammation and lymphoid organ development. The mechanisms of these processes are most likely quite similar and involve adhesion molecules and chemokines. They produce entities, the lymphoid organs and the inflammatory sites, with comparable functions, namely antigen presentation and T- and B-cell reactivity. In the case of an invading pathogen, this contributes to defense. In the case of an autoimmune reaction, it leads to exacerbation through determinant spreading.

Acknowledgments
These studies were supported by NIH grant RO1 CA 16885 and a grant from the National Multiple Sclerosis Society RG 2394. I acknowledge the intellectual and experimental input of Peter Hjelmstrom, Cheryl Bergman, Myriam Hill, Amy Juedes, Rosalba Sacca, and Carolyn Cuff.

References

1   Cuff CA, Ruddle NH (1998) Lymphotoxin. In: PJ Delves, I Roitt (eds): *Encyclopedia of immunology*. Academic Press, London, 1637–1641

2   Kratz A, Campos-Neto A, Hanson MS, Ruddle NH (1996) Chronic inflammation caused by lymphotoxin is lymphoid neogenesis. *J Exp Med* 183: 1461–1472

3   Lehmann PV, Sercarz EE, Forsthuber T, Dayan CM, Gammon G (1993) Determinant spreading and the dynamics of the autoimmune T-cell repertoire. *Immunol Today* 14: 203–208

4   Cuff CA, Schwartz J, Bergman C, Russell KS, Bender JR, Ruddle NH (1998) Lymphotoxin alpha3 induces chemokines and adhesion moleulces: Insight into the role of LT alpha in inflammation and lymphoid organ development. *J Immunol* 161: 6853–6860

5   Sacca R, Cuff CA, Ruddle NH (1997) Mediators of inflammation. *Curr Opin Immunol* 9: 851–857

6   Powell MB, Mitchell D, Lederman J, Buckmeier J, Zamvil SS, Graham M, Ruddle NH, Steinman L (1990) Lymphotoxin and tumor necrosis factor-alpha production by myelin basic protein-specific T cell clones correlates with encephalitogenicity. *International Immunol* 2: 539–544

7   Santambrogio L, Hochwald GM, Saxena B, Leu CH, Martz JE, Carlino JA, Ruddle NH, Palladino MA, Gold LI, Thorbecke GJ (1993) Studies on the mechanisms by which TGF-β protects against allergic encephalomyelitis: antagonism between TGF-β and TNF. *J Immunol* 151: 1116–1127

8   Ruddle NH, Bergman CM, McGrath KM, Lingenheld EG, Grunnet ML, Padula SJ, Clark RB (1990) An antibody to lymphotoxin and tumor necrosis factor prevents transfer of experimental allergic encephalomyelitis. *J Exp Med* 172: 1193–1200

9   Selmaj K, Raine CS, Cross AH (1991) Anti-tumor necrosis factor therapy abrogates autoimmune demyelination. *Ann Neurol* 30: 694–700

10   Selmaj K, Papierz W, Glabinski A, Kohno T (1995) Prevention of chronic relapsing experimental autoimmune encephalomyelitis by soluble tumor necrosis factor receptor I. *J Neuroimmun* 56: 135–141

11   Suen WE, Bergman CM, Hjelmstrom P, Ruddle NH (1997) A critical role for lymphotoxin in experimental allergic encephalomyelitis. *J Exp Med* 186: 1233–1240

12   Hjelmstrom P, Juedes AE, Ruddle NH (1998) Cytokines and antibodies in oligodendrocyte glycoprotein-induced experimental allergic encephalomyelitis. In: *Research in Immunology*, vol. 75. Publications Scientifiques, Paris, 42–52

13   Selmaj K, Raine CF, Farooq M, Norton WT, Brosnan CF (1991) Cytokine cytotoxicity against oligodendrocytes: Apoptosis induced by lymphotoxin. *J Immunol* 147: 1522–1529

14   Koni PA, Sacca R, Lawton P, Browning JL, Ruddle NH, Flavell RA (1997) Distinct roles in lymphoid organogenesis for lymphotoxins alpha and beta revealed in lymphotoxin beta-deficient mice. *Immunity* 6: 491–500

15   Hjelmstrom P, Juedes AE, Fjell J, Ruddle NH (1998) Cutting edge: B cell-deficient mice develop experimental allergic encephalomyelitis with demyelination after myelin oligodendrocuyte glycoprotein sensitization. *J Immunol* 161: 4480–4483

16   Eugster H-P, Frei K, Kopf M, Lassmann H, Fontana A (1998) IL-6 deficient mice resist

myelin oligodendrocyte glycoprotein-induced autoimmune encephalomyelitis. *Eur J Immunol* 28: 2178–2187

17 Barten DM, Ruddle NH (1994) Vascular cell adhesion molecule-1 modulation by TNF in experimental allergic encephalomyeleits. *J Neuroimmunol* 51: 123–133

18 Picarella DE, Kratz A, Li C-b, Ruddle NH, Flavell RA (1992) Insulitis in transgenic mice expressing TNF-β (lymphotoxin) in the pancreas. *Proc Natl Acad Sci* 89: 10036–10040

19 Sacca R, Turley S, Soong L, Mellman I, Ruddle NH (1997) Transgenic expression of lymphotoxin restores lymph nodes to lymphotoxin-α deficient mice. *J Immunol* 159: 4252–4260

Chemokine/cytokine biology during the evolution of fibrotic disease

Steven L. Kunkel, Sem H. Phan, Nicholas W. Lukacs, Cory Hogaboam and Stephen W. Chensue

Department of Pathology, University of Michigan Medical School, 5214, Med Sci I, 1301 Catherine Rd, Ann Arbor, MI 48109-0602, USA

Introduction

Although the sequence of events in the pathology of many interstitial fibrotic diseases is not well characterized, numerous factors that regulate immune and fibrotic processes have been implicated in the evolution of these disorders. These processes include potential viral infections [1], genetic variations [2], immune complexes [3], environmental factors [4] and effector cell activation [5]. This last category has generated recent interest, as the classification of effector cells can no longer be limited to peripheral blood leukocytes, but must include resident stromal and parenchymal cells that comprise the tissue. Epithelial cells [6], endothelial cells [7], and fibroblasts[8] have all been identified as effector cells *via* their ability to generate significant levels of regulatory cytokines and chemokines that participate in cytokine networks. Of particular interest is the elevated levels of chemokines that these non-inflammatory cells can express when activated. Table 1 contains representative ligands and their corresponding receptors for the CC and CXC chemokine families. This list is not inclusive as it is now known that there are at least four supergene families of chemokines containing over 50 different proteins.

The participation of nonimmune cells in the lung to the evolution of interstitial disease is more diverse than simply serving as a passive target, leading to injury, as these cells contribute to the pathogenesis of fibrotic disease. For example, fibroblasts are critical to the evolution of interstitial fibrotic disease, as these cells can synthesize both cytokines, chemokines, and extracellular matrix. While the processes which lead to an increase in extracellular matrix deposition are not totally clear, it is apparent that inflammatory/immune cells, cytokines, and activated stromal cells themselves are contributing factors to end-stage disease [9]. Moreover, it is likely that cytokine networks are ultimately responsible for cell-to-cell communication which dictates the progression of chronic inflammation leading to fibrosis.

Inflammatory Processes: Molecular Mechanisms and Therapeutic Opportunities, edited by L. Gordon Letts and Douglas W. Morgan
© 2000 Birkhäuser Verlag Basel/Switzerland

Table 1 - Most of the chemokines discovered to date belong to either the CXC or CC super-gene family. This table contains representative members of CC and CXC chemokine ligands and their receptors.

CC chemokines		CXC chemokines	
Receptor	Ligand	Receptor	Ligand
CCR1	MIP-1α, RANTES	CXCR1	IL-8
CCR2	MCP-1,2,3	CXCR2	(promiscuous) CXC
CCR3	Eotaxin, RANTES, MCP-3	CXCR3	MIG, IP10
CCR4	MIP-1α, RANTES	CXCR4	SDF-1
CCR5	MIP-1α,β, RANTES	CXCR5	B cell attracting chemokine-1
CCR6	LARC		
CCR7	ELC		
CCR8	I 309		
CCR9	MCP-1, MCP-3		

Cytokines, chemokines and chronic inflammation leading to fibrosis

A variety of cytokines and chemokines have been found associated with chronic inflammation and fibrosis, including interleukin-1 (IL-1) [10], interleukin-6 (IL-6) [11], interleukin-8 (IL-8) [12], macrophage inflammatory protein-1α (MIP-1α) [13], monocyte chemoattractant protein-1 (MCP-1) [14], tumor necrosis factor (TNF) [15], transforming growth factors [16], granulocyte-macrophage colony stimulating factor (GM-CSF) [17], macrophage-CSF (M-CSF) [17], and platelet-derived growth factor (PDGF) [18]. This list contains representative cytokines which possess early activation, chemotactic, growth and differentiation, and remodeling activity (Tab. 2). For example, TGFβ possesses a number of activities that would suggest a profibrotic role in lung disease. TGFβ directly increases the gene expression of extracellular matrix molecules by stromal cells, inhibits collagenase production, and influences fibroblast proliferation via the induction of fibroblast growth factors [16].

The identification of different cytokines from either patients with sarcoidosis or idiopathic pulmonary fibrosis or animal models that mimic human fibrosis have provided clues that specific immune mediators are involved in the evolution of interstitial disease. However, a causal role of these cytokines in the initiation and maintenance of chronic inflammation has not been clearly established. Thus, the biomedical community is still far from understanding the mechanisms which dictate either the restoration of normal lung tissue or the progression to irreversible fibrot-

Table 2 - Specific cytokines participate in the evolution of an inflammatory response as it matures from the initiation stage (early activation and chemotactic), through the maintenance stage (chemotactic and differentiation), and finally the resolution phase (remodeling).

Inflammatory event	Cytokine
Early activation	IL-1, TNF
Chemotactic	Chemokines
Differentiation	IFNγ
Remodeling	TGFβ, FGF

ic derangements. However, there is a growing body of scientific evidence suggesting that the cytokine profile of the natural immune/inflammatory response likely determines the disease phenotype responsible for either resolution or progression to end-stage fibrosis.

Much of the supporting evidence is derived from studies demonstrating that interferons, especially interferon γ (IFNγ), have profound suppressive effects on the production of such extracellular matrix proteins as collagen and fibronectin. Investigations have demonstrated that interferons can inhibit both fibroblast and chondrocyte collagen production *in vitro*, as well as decrease the expression of steady-state type I and III procollagen mRNA levels in these cells. In addition, the administration of IFNγ *in vivo* can cause a reduction of extracellular matrix in animal models of fibrosis. This information supports the concept that IFNγ, one of the major Th1 type cytokines, possesses profound regulatory activity for collagen deposition during chronic inflammation. Interestingly, interleukin-4 (IL-4), one of the major Th2 type cytokines, is a potent stimulus for the production of fibroblast-derived extracellular matrix, including type I and III collagen and fibronectin [19]. These studies have demonstrated that IL-4 treatment of fibroblasts can increase steady-state levels of extracellular matrix mRNA and subsequent production of extracellular matrix protein. In addition, IL-4 has been identified as a chemotactic factor for directed movement of fibroblasts [20]. These studies lend support to the theory that the disease phenotype characterized by either Th1 or Th2 like cytokines may be paramount in determining the course of chronic inflammation, leading to interstitial fibrosis.

Functional activity of type 1 and type 2 cytokines

There is abundant evidence supporting the paradigm that the initiation, maintenance, and resolution of immune reactivity is governed by a complex network of cytokines [21]. However, much of our knowledge regarding the potential mechanisms whereby cytokines function in the various phases of an immune response are derived from *in vitro* studies that are often difficult to translate into *in vivo* inflammatory events. This concern is further compounded by the heterogeneity of cytokines and inflammatory responses that can be observed under different clinical conditions. The discovery by Mosmann and colleagues that T-helper cell subsets could be classified on the basis of cytokine profiles has provided a degree of clarification to chronic cell mediated immune responses [22]. The Th1 and Th2 cytokine patterns were originally identified from a panel of T-helper cell clones and include IFNγ and IL-2 *versus* IL-4, IL-5, and IL-10, respectively. IFNγ and IL-12 are now particularly noted for their role in delayed type hypersensitivity reactions, while IL-4, IL-5, and IL-10 are important in B-cell activation and antibody production. Evidence from both experimental models and human studies suggests that the balance between Th1 and Th2 cytokines are important in determining the state of resistance to certain infections.

For example, resistance to intracellular pathogens such as *Mycobacteria* and *Leishmania* sp. depends upon an effective Th1 cytokine response, while a Th2 cytokine response seems to negate this resistant state [23, 24]. In general terms, immune responses dominated by IFNγ are especially important in clearing intracellular infectious agents, while those immune responses characterized by IL-4, IL-5, and IL-10 would appear to be most important in extracellular infections where an antibody response would be efficacious. In addition, the balance of Th1 and Th2 cytokines has been attributed to the phenomenon of cross-regulation. Specifically, IFNγ promotes the differentiation of Th1 cells, while IL-4 and IL-10 appear to shift immune responses to a Th2 like pattern by promoting both Th2 cell differentiation and suppressing Th1 cell activity [25]. *In vitro* studies have further demonstrated cross-regulation in that IL-10 and IL-4 can inhibit the production of IL-12, whereas IFNγ can augment the expression of this Th1 cytokine [26].

Type 2 cytokines are associated with cell-mediated inflammation and fibroblast activation

Some of the most common world-wide diseases which are dominated by Th2 cytokines and eventual end-stage fibrosis of target tissue are helminth parasitic infections [27]. For example, schistosomiasis is one of the world's most prevalent forms of chronic cell-mediated inflammation and possesses a cytokine phenotype characterized by high levels of IL-4, IL-5, and IL-10, with corresponding low levels of IFNγ [27]. In addition, the fibrotic response of the host during this disease greatly contributes to the morbidity associated with the parasitic infection. The vigorous fibrotic response to the schistosome egg granuloma is the consequence of a parasite-induced, host-derived cytokine profile which likely allows the parasite to survive, while effectively fibrosing or "walling off" the deposited parasite egg. Interestingly, the treatment of murine schistosomiasis with exogenous IFNγ significantly decreases collagen deposition associated with granuloma formation. These studies lend support to the potential disparate role of Th1 and Th2 cytokines during the evolution of fibrotic processes. The opposing effects of Th1 and Th2 cytokines in fibrosis are further supported by a number of recent investigations demonstrating that IL-4 is an important mediator of fibroblast activation [19, 20].

These studies have shown that IL-4 can induce fibroblast proliferation, cytokine synthesis, and extracellular matrix production. Interestingly, the intensity of IL-4-induced fibroblast collagen synthesis was of the same order of magnitude as that induced by equal amounts of TGFβ. Additional studies have also identified that IL-4 can effectively communicate with fibroblasts *via* a single class of high affinity IL-4 receptors [28]. Fibroblasts possess both a membrane bound form of the IL-4 receptor, as well as a secreted form of the IL-4 receptor. The soluble IL-4 receptor is derived from a truncation of the membrane form and may serve as either an IL-4 binding protein with antagonist activity or as a carrier of IL-4 with its biological properties left intact. A more thorough assessment of fibroblasts has identified that these cells likely reside in the interstitium as a heterogeneous pool of cells. In addition, these studies have shown that recovered murine lung fibroblasts can be separated into two functionally and morphologically distinct subsets which express different levels of IL-4 receptors on their surface and respond to IL-4 in a diverse manner. The above information underscores the pleiotropic activities of IL-4, as fibroblast activation must be included on the list of activities along with the proliferation of B cells, T lymphocytes, mast cells and hematopoietic progenitor cells.

While there is little doubt that Th2 cytokines may predominate in specific parasitic infections, interesting data have recently accumulated suggesting that certain cell mediated responses have characteristic Th2 cytokine profiles [29]. Murine models of chronic graft-vs-host disease, as a result of experimental bone marrow transplant, have been characterized by a hypergammaglobulinemia, high levels of IgE, immune complex deposition in tissues, and elevated concentrations of IL-4. When mice with bone marrow transplant-graft-vs-host disease were treated with neutralizing IL-4 antibodies, IgE levels dropped, immune complex-induced lesions resolved, and splenomegaly was prevented. Interestingly, cyclosporine A, an agent known to suppress Th1 cytokine responses, caused an exacerbation of bone marrow transplant graft-vs-host disease in these models [30]. While clinical studies assessing longitudinal alterations in cytokine levels and corresponding changes in lung pathology are difficult to perform in human bone marrow transplants with subsequent graft-vs-host disease, it is known that fibrosis and subsequent cell proliferation associated with bronchiolitis obliterans may be a consequence of the transplant.

One of the more compelling pieces of information which may link the expression of Th2 cytokines to the evolution of fibrosis is the association of fibroblast activation and the presence of eosinophils [31]. A number of studies have demonstrated that asthma and parasitic infections are associated with both Th2 cytokine expression (IL-4 and IL-5) and a profound eosinophilia, as IL-5 is both an eosinophilopoeitic and chemotactic factor for eosinophils [32]. While the mechanistic role of eosinophils and Th2 cytokines has been demonstrated in asthma and parasitic infections, the role of these cells and Th2 cytokines in other disease states is not as clear. However, recent data have demonstrated an eosinophilia in disorders in which fibrosis occurs [33]. In addition, *in vitro* experiments have shown that eosinophils are capable of a time-dependent release of factors which stimulate human fibroblasts to undergo replication and synthesize extracellular matrix [34]. The interactions between fibroblasts and eosinophils appear to be rather complex, as fibroblast conditioned media has also been shown to prolong the survival of eosinophils. Nonetheless, studies have identified an increase in eosinophils in association with fibrotic changes in idiopathic pulmonary fibrosis [33]. Thus, a potential fibrotic network, leading to end-stage pathology, may be established between the triumvirate of type 2 cytokines, eosinophils, and fibroblasts.

Animal models of interstitial lung disease possess specific phenotypes

Information derived from a variety of experimental animal models suggests that a number of cytokines play a role in the initiation, maintenance, and resolution of chronic interstitial inflammation. However, the likely mechanism for each cytokine during the evolution of the inflammatory response has only recently been addressed. For example, *in vivo* studies assessing the development of interstitial lung granulomas induced by mycobacterial antigen have demonstrated that gamma-IFN and TNF were necessary cytokines for lesion progression [35]. In contrast, pulmonary inflammation initiated by embolization of *Schistosoma mansoni* eggs was maintained by IL-4 [36]. These cytokine profiles suggest that interstitial delayed-type hypersensitivity granulomatous inflammation involves Th1 and/or Th2 cytokines. In the context of interstitial lung inflammation, these observations served as the basis for the establishment of models that exhibit either a Th1 or Th2 inflammatory response within the lung. This was accomplished by presensitization of mice with *Mycobacteria* species (BCG) or *Schistosoma mansoni* eggs followed by pulmonary embolization of Sephadex (carbohydrate beads) coated with a known amount of soluble antigen, purified protein derivative (PPD) or schistosome egg antigen (SEA), derived from the respective organisms [35]. The two types of lung lesions have distinctive histological characteristics. The Th1 response contained mostly small and large mononuclear cells, whereas the Th2 lesion contained both mononuclear cells and a significant number of eosinophils. In the resolution phase the Th2 response was more cellular than the Th1 response and was associated with a substantial increase in the number of fibroblasts. While these models have been used to investigate leukocyte recruitment in the lung, they have not been utilized to address the mechanism of progressive pulmonary fibrosis. The use of clearly defined Th1 and Th2 lung models will prove important in understanding the cellular and molecular regulation of fibroblast activation and interstitial fibrosis that accompanies these specific responses.

The role of chemokines in fibroblast activation and fibrosis

A variety of studies have identified the potential role of specific chemokines in the elicitation of blood borne leukocytes. Interestingly, the elevation of chemokines, such as MCP-1, has not always correlated with the infiltration of mononuclear leukocytes. This suggests that other biological activities may be associated with the expression of MCP-1 independent of leukocyte recruitement. The ability of fibroblast to generate significant levels of MCP-1 served as an impetus to determine if fibroblast generated MCP-1 could serve as a potential autocrine or paracrine activator of fibroblasts. Thus, primary cultures of isolated fibroblasts were treated with increasing doses of MCP-1 for different periods of time and assessed for the production of procollagen type I mRNA. These studies demonstrated that MCP-1, over a 24-h time span, was able to stimulate collagen expression in a dose-dependent manner [37].

It is a well known phenomenon that cytokine induce their cellular effects *via* engaging cytokine networks, thus, additional studies were conducted to identified other distal mediators that may have been up-regulated by MCP-1. One of the key cytokines that is known to activate fibroblasts is transforming growth factor-beta (TGF) and antibodies to this reparative cytokine was found to inhibit MCP-1-induced collagen expression. Furthermore, pretreatment of the fibroblasts with antisense TGF oligodeoxyribonucleotides inhibited the ability of MCP-1 to increase the expression of collagen mRNA. These studies demonstrate the MCP-1 has a novel effect on fibroblast activation *via* augmenting the production of TGF which in turn increases the production of fibroblast derived collagen. These studies have important implication regarding a unique role for chemokines in the reparative or end-stage phase of chronic inflammation.

Acknowledgements
This work was supported in part by NIH grants: HL-31963, HL 35276, P50HL56402, IP50HL46487.

References

1   Patchefsky AS, Banner M, Freundlich IM (1971) Desquamative interstitial pneumonia: Significance of intranuclear viral-like inclusion bodies. *Ann Intern Med* 74: 322–327

2   Bitterman PB, Rennard SI, Keogh BA, Wewers MD, Adelberg S, Crystal RG (1984) Familial idiopathic pulmonary fibrosis: Evidence of lung inflammation in unaffected family members. *N Eng J Med* 314: 1343–1347

3   Nagaya H, Elmore M, Ford CD (1973) Idiopathic pulmonary fibrosis: An immune complex disease? *Am Rev Respir Dis* 107: 826–830

4   Rom WN, Travis WD, Brody AR (1991) Cellular and molecular basis of the asbestos-related diseases. *Am Rev Respir Dis* 143: 408–422

5   Kallenberg CGM, Schilizzi BM, Beaumont F, DeLeij L, Poppema S (1987) Expression of cell II major histocompatibility complex antigen on alveolar epithelium in interstitial lung disease: Relevance to pathogenesis of idiopathic pulmonary fibrosis. *J Clin Pathol* 40: 725–733

6   Standiford TJ, Kunkel SL, Phan SH, Rollins BJ, Strieter RM (1991) Alveolar macrophage-derived cytokines induce monocyte chemoattractant protein-1 expression from human pulmonary type II-like epithelial cells. *J Biol Chem* 266: 9912–9918

7   Strieter RM, Kunkel SL, Showell HJ, Remick DG, Phan SH, Ward PA, Marks RM (1989) Endothelial cell gene expression of a neutrophil chemotactic factor by TNFα, LPS, and IL-1β. *Science* 243: 1467–1469

8   Rolfe MW, Kunkel SL, Standiford TJ, Orringer MB, Phan SH, Evanoff HL, Burdick MD, Strieter RM (1992) Expression and regulation of human pulmonary fibroblast-derived monocyte chemotactic peptide (MCP-1). *Am J Physiol: Lung Cell Molec Physiol* 263: 536–545

9   Phan SH, Kunkel SL (1992) Lung cytokine production in bleomycin-induced pulmonary fibrosis. *Exp Lung Res* 18: 29–43

10 Chensue SW, Ottrness IG, Higashi GI, Forch C, Kunkel SL (1989) Monokine production by hypersensitivity (*Schistosoma mansoni* egg) and foreign body (Sephadex bead)-type granuloma macrophages. Evidence for sequential production of IL-1 and TNF. *J Immunol* 142: 1281–1286

11 Sibille Y, Houssiau F, Pochet JM, Staquet P, Van Snick J, Van Leuven F (1990) Alpha 2 macroglobulin and Interleukin-6 release by human alveolar macrophages from normal and sarcoidosis patients. *Am Rev Resp Dis* 141: A8712

12 Lynch JP, Standiford TJ, Rolfe MW, Kunkel SL, Strieter RM (1992) Neutrophilic alveolitis in idiopathic pulmonary fibrosis. The role of interleukin-8. *Am Rev Res Dis* 145: 1433–1439

13 Lukacs NW, Kunkel SL, Strieter RM, Warmington K, Chensue SW (1993) The role of macrophage inflammatory protein 1 alpha in *Schistosoma mansoni* egg-induced granulomatous inflammation. *J Exp Med* 177: 1551–1559

14 Chensue SL, Warmington KS, Lukacs NW, Lincoln PM, Burdick MD, Strieter RM, Kunkel SL (1995) Monocyte chemotactic protein (MCP-1) expression during schisto-

some egg granuloma formation: Sequence of production, localization, contribution, and regulation. *Am J Pathol* 146: 130–138

15   Bachwich PR, Lynch JP, Larrick J, Spengler M, Kunkel SL (1986) Tumor necrosis factor production by human sarcoid alveolar macrophages. *Am J Pathol* 125: 421–425

16   Khalil N, Bereznay O, Sporin M, Greenberg AH (1989) Macrophage production of TGF-beta and fibroblast collagen synthesis in chronic pulmonary fibrosis. *J Exp Med* 170: 727–737

17   Gauldie J, Jordana M, Cox G (1993) Cytokines and pulmonary fibrosis. *Thorax* 48: 931–935

18   Bonner JC, Osornio-Vargas AR, Badgett A, Brody AR (1991) Differential proliferation of rat lung fibroblasts induced by the platelet-derived growth factor-AA, AB, and BB isoforms secreted by alveolar macrophages. *Am J Respir Cell Mol Biol* 5: 539–547

19   Postlewaite AE, Holness MA, Katai H, Raghow R (1992) Human fibroblasts synthesize elevated levels of extracellular matrix proteins in response to interleukin-4. *J Clin Invest* 90: 1479–1485

20   Postlewaite AE, Seyer JM. (1991) Fibroblast chemotaxis induction by human recombinant interleukin-4. *J Clin Invest* 87: 2147–2152

21   Chensue SW, Warmington KS, Ruth J, Lincoln PM, Kunkel SL (1994) Cross-regulatory role of interferon-gamma (IFNγ), IL-4 and IL-10 in schistosome egg granuloma formation: *in vivo* regulation of Th activity and inflammation. *Clin Exp Immunol* 98: 395–400

22   Mosmann TRH, Cherwinski H, Bond MW (1986) Two types of murine T cell clones. I. Definition according to profiles of lymphokine activity and secreted proteins. *J Immunol* 136: 2348–2357

23   Yamamura MK, Uyemura RJ, Deans K, Weinberg TH, Rea BR, Bloom BR, Modlin RL (1991) Defining protective responses to pathogens: cytokine profiles in leprosy lesions. *Science* 254: 277–281

24   Chatelain RK, Varkila K, Coffman RL (1992) IL-4 induces a Th2 response in Leishmania major-infected mice. *J Immunol* 148: 1182–1194

25   Swain SL, Weinberg AD, English M, Huston G (1990) IL-4 and IFN direct the development of distinct subsets of helper T cells. *Fed Proc* 4: 2020

26   Trinchieri G, Scott P (1994) The role of interleukin-12 in the immune response, disease and therapy. *Immunol Today* 15: 460–467

27   Chensue SW, Warmington Ruth JH, Lincoln P, Kunkel S (1995) Cytokine function during mycobacterial and schistosomal antigen-induced pulmonary granuloma formation. Local and regional participation of IFN, IL-10 and TNF. *J Immunol* 154: 5969–5976

28   Sempowski GD, Beckmann MP, Derdak S, Phipps RP (1994) Subsets of murine lung fibroblasts express membrane-bound and soluble IL-4 receptors. *J Immunol* 152: 3606–3614

29   Goldman M, Druet D, Gleichmann E (1991) Th2 cells in systemic autoimmunity; insights from allogeneic disease and chemically-induced autoimmunity. *Immunol Today* 12: 223–228

30 Glazier A, Tutschka J, Farmer ER, Santos GW (1983) Graft-vs-host disease in cyclosporin rats after syngeneic and autologous bone marrow reconstitution. *J Exp Med* 158: 1–13

31 Weller PA (1989) Eosinophils and fibroblasts: The medium in the mesenchyme. *Am J Resp Cell Mol Biol* 1: 267–268

32 OwenWF, Rothenberg ME, Peterson J, Weller PF, Silberstein D, Sheffer AL, Stevens RL, Soberman RJ, Austen KF (1988) Interleukin-5 and phenotypically altered eosinophils in the blood of patients with idiopathic hypereosinophilic syndrome. *J Exp Med* 170: 343–355

33 Peterson MW, Monick M, Hunninghake GW (1987) Prognostic role of eosinophils in pulmonary fibrosis. *Chest* 92: 51–56

34 Shock A, Rabe F, Dent G, Chambers RC, Gray AJ, Chung KF, Barnes PJ, Laurent GJ (1991) Eosinophils adhere to and stimulate replication of lung fibroblasts *in vitro*. *Clin Exp Immunol* 86: 185–190

35 Chensue SW, Warmington K, Ruth J, Lincoln P, Kuo MC, Kunkel SL (1994) Cytokine responses during mycobacterial and schistosomal antigen-induced pulmonary granuloma formation. Production of Th1 and Th2 cytokines and relative contribution of TNF. *Am J Pathol* 145: 1105–1114

36 Chensue SW, Terebuh PD, Warmington K, Hershey SD, Evanoff HL, Kunkel SL, Higashi GI (1992) Role of IL-4 and IFN-gamma in *Schistosoma mansoni* egg-induced hypersensitivity granuloma formation. *J Immunol* 148: 900–910

37 Gharaee-Kermani M, Denholm EM, Phan SM (1996) Costimulation of fibroblast collagen and transforming growth factor Beta gene expression by monocyte chemoattractant protein-1 via specific receptors. *J Biol Chem* 271: 17779–17784

The role of MCP-1 in disease

Long Gu, Susan C. Tseng, and Barrett J. Rollins

Department of Adult Oncology, Dana-Farber Cancer Institute, Harvard Medical School, 44 Binney Street, Boston, MA 02115, USA

Introduction

Monocyte chemoattractant protein-1 (MCP-1), also known as monocyte chemotactic and activating factor (MCAF), is a CC chemokine that exerts its effects specifically on monocytes, memory T lymphocytes, NK cells, and basophils. Originally cloned as the murine *JE* gene on the basis of its growth factor-inducible expression [1, 2], the protein was later purified as a monocyte-specific chemoattractant [3-5]. While most chemokines bind to multiple receptors, suggesting that the chemokine system may be plagued by biological redundancy, the sole receptor for MCP-1 identified to date is CCR2 [6]. Like other chemokine receptors, CCR2 is a seven trans-membrane spanning receptor coupled predominantly to $G_{i\alpha}$, although there is evidence for coupling to other G protein subtypes as well [7].

Structure/activity relationships for MCP-1 have been explored using site-directed mutagenesis. As with CXC chemokines, the N-terminal domain of MCP-1 is essential for activity as are some amino acids in the loop between cysteine-2 and cysteine-3 [8, 9]. Also important are selected residues in the β-pleated sheets that form the Greek key motif found in all chemokines. Some of the variants created for these analyses have potent MCP-1 inhibitory properties. In particular, N-terminally truncated variants known as 7ND and MCP-1 9–76 can inhibit MCP-1-mediated monocyte chemotaxis [8–10]. The mechanism of action of these inhibitors is controversial. On one hand, they may simply compete with MCP-1 for binding to CCR2. On the other hand, since MCP-1 forms dimers, they may act as dominant negative inhibitors [10].

One of the main reasons for interest in MCP-1 is that its expression has been documented in a variety of diseases characterized by mononuclear cell infiltration. Several of these are listed in Table 1. The presence of MCP-1 in these diseases leads to the hypothesis that MCP-1 is responsible for their inflammatory components. Testing this hypothesis has been a critically important endeavor in chemokine research since a demonstration of MCP-1's importance in disease would validate

Inflammatory Processes: Molecular Mechanisms and Therapeutic Opportunities, edited by L. Gordon Letts and Douglas W. Morgan
© 2000 Birkhäuser Verlag Basel/Switzerland

Table 1 - Expression of MCP-1 in non-infectious disease

Atherosclerosis (experimental and human)
Rheumatoid arthritis
Asthma
Multiple Sclerosis (and EAE)
Alzheimer's Disease
Idiopathic Pulmonary Fibrosis
Glomerulonephritis

MCP-1 and CCR2 as drug targets. This chapter describes some of the recent results that confirm an essential and non-redundant role for these molecules in a variety of diseases.

MCP-1's activities *in vivo*

Prior to examining MCP-1's role in disease, it was essential to show that MCP-1 actually attracts monocytes *in vivo*. Without such a demonstration, it would remain possible that MCP-1's ability to attract monocytes or T lymphocytes in Boyden chambers *in vitro* would not accurately predict its *in vivo* functions. The easiest test of MCP-1 function *in vivo* consists of injecting purified MCP-1 into rodent skin and monitoring the presence of infiltrating leukocytes. In some of the original descriptions of purified human MCP-1, data were presented that injection of this material into mouse skin elicited a monocyte-rich infiltrate [11]. However, it was also reported that large amounts of recombinant murine MCP-1 produced no convincing infiltration after intradermal injection [12].

To address this controversy, several groups developed transgenic mouse models in which MCP-1 expression was driven by a variety of tissue-specific promoters. The earliest model used the mouse mammary tumor virus long terminal repeat (MMTV-LTR) to target the expression of murine MCP-1 to a variety of organs including breast, gonads, salivary gland, lung, and kidney [13]. Despite achieving high levels of expression in these organs, no mononuclear infiltrates were noted. This was most likely due to the fact that these mice had high serum levels of MCP-1 which were either desensitizing MCP-1 receptors on circulating monocytes or canceling the chemoattractant concentration gradient emanating from the expressing organs. Nonetheless, the mice were more susceptible to lethal infection by intracellular pathogens such as *L. monocytogenes* and *M. tuberculosis*, suggesting that MCP-1 plays a role in host resistance to these organisms.

Since then, other transgenic mice have been constructed that use promoters with more localized and lower levels of expression. For example, one group has targeted murine MCP-1 expression to thymus and brain using the lck and myelin basic protein (MBP) promoters, respectively [14]. In the lck model, a low level monocytic infiltrate in the thymus was detected by flow cytometry. In the MBP model, perivascular cuffing of monocytes around brain vessels could be observed during the postnatal period during which the MBP promoter is active. The number of infiltrating cells and their depth within the brain parenchyma could be enhanced by systemic administration of lipopolysaccharide.

Another model used the keratin-14 promoter to direct murine MCP-1 expression to the skin [15]. A subtle phenotype induced by the transgene appeared to involve an increased number of dendritic cells in the dermis. In addition, however, these mice displayed an exaggerated contact hypersensitivity response compared to wild type animals. Presumably, constitutive MCP-1 expression was able to enhance either the afferent or efferent arm, or perhaps both, of the hypersensitivity response.

A fourth model directed human MCP-1 expression to the lung using a surfactant promoter [16]. In this case, increased numbers of mononuclear cells were recovered in the bronchoalveolar lavage, but infiltration into the pulmonary parenchyma *per se* was not observed. However, embolizing yeast cell wall glucan to the lung produced granulomata that were more cellular in the transgenic mice. Notably, this transgene used human MCP-1 to elicit responses in mice, suggesting that cross-species models may have some utility in drug discovery.

A fifth model examined the consequences of cardiac expression of murine MCP-1 by using the α-cardiac myosin heavy chain promoter [17]. This produced a monocytic infiltrate into the myocardium that resulted in cardiac hypertrophy and dilation. Thus deregulated expression of a single gene product can produce myocarditis and cardiomyopathy.

Finally, murine MCP-1 expression controlled by the insulin promoter resulted in a monocytic insulitis [18]. However, despite the presence of a lifelong infiltrate, the mice never became diabetic. These mice were mated to the MMTV transgenic mice described above, and mice that inherited both transgenes showed no infiltrates despite expressing the same amount of MCP-1 in the pancreas as mice that inherited only the insulin promoter transgene. This confirmed the presumption that high levels of circulating MCP-1 could prevent monocytes from responding to low levels of locally produced MCP-1.

Taken together, the data from transgenic mouse models permit several inferences. First, it is clear that MCP-1 can attract monocytes *in vivo*. Second, in none of these models were T lymphocytes observed despite MCP-1's potent T-lymphocytic chemoattractant properties *in vitro*. This is most likely due to the fact that CCR2 expression is not constitutive in T cells but must be induced. Third, in all models except the α-cardiac myosin mouse, little or no tissue destruction occurred despite the presence of monocytes. This suggests that, in general, MCP-1 is designed to attract monocytes without necessarily activating them, and that second signals are required to engage monocyte effector functions.

MCP-1's role in inflammation and the immune response

The cleanest approach to determining whether or not MCP-1 plays a non-redundant role in physiology is a genetic one. Both *MCP-1* and *CCR2* have been genetically deleted in mice, and a variety of experiments have documented the importance of this ligand/receptor pair in inflammation and the immune response. For example, instilling thioglycollate broth into the peritoneum of a mouse results 72 h later in a macrophage-rich peritonitis. In the absence of MCP-1 or CCR2, a small number of neutrophils and eosinophils can be found in the peritoneum in numbers similar to those in wild type animals [19–22]. However, there is no increase in macrophages in the knockout animals. Thus CCR2 activation is required for monocyte elicitation in this model and the only ligand of CCR2 that is relevant is MCP-1. Similar defects in the absence of CCR2 were observed in a model of yeast β-glucan granuloma formation [22] and after challenge with *L. monocytogenes* [21].

In models of delayed type hypersensitivity (DTH), the vasogenic swelling response is intact in MCP-1-deficient mice [19]. However, the number of macrophages recruited to the challenge site is decreased by 60% in the absence of MCP-1, indicating a non-redundant role for MCP-1 in monocyte recruitment in this specific immune response. Along the same lines, both in MCP-1-deficient mice and in mice treated with anti-MCP-1 antibodies, fewer cells are recruited to granulomata induced by the eggs of *S. mansoni* when they are embolized in the pulmonary vasculature [19]. This only occurs in mice already sensitized to *Schistosoma* egg antigen, and the response has a number of characteristics suggesting that it is driven by Th2 cells. This would indicate that MCP-1 either drives or is part of the effector arm of a Th2 response. Consistent with that notion is the observation that naïve T cells can be stimulated to differentiate along a Th2 pathway *in vitro* by treating them with MCP-1 [23].

In contrast, it has been reported that CCR2-deficient mice have a Th1 defect [20]. This was based on the observation that PPD-sensitized mice recruited fewer cells to pulmonary granulomata induced by embolization of PPD-coated beads, which is predominantly a Th1 response. Furthermore, cells from draining lymph nodes in the PPD-bead-challenged knockout mice secreted almost no interferon-γ (IFNγ) while wild type mice secreted large amounts.

It is not clear why MCP-1-deficient mice appear to have defective Th2 responses while CCR2-deficient mice have Th1 defects. One possibility is that in the absence of MCP-1, the other four ligands for CCR2 exert an effect that induces Th1 responses in a normal way. Alternatively, these experiments have been performed in hybrid mice, and it may be that once the disrupted alleles are placed in homogeneous genetic backgrounds, other results may be observed. Regardless of the explanation, these models indicate that in addition to having an influence on cell recruitment in inflammation, MCP-1 also has an effect on T-helper cell differentiation.

MCP-1 in disease models

Three experimental approaches have been taken to examining MCP-1's role in disease models, namely antibody neutralization, administration of antagonists, and genetic deletion of MCP-1 and its receptor, CCR2. Since microbial infections would be expected to induce chemokine expression to recruit leukocytes, the following discussion will be restricted to disease models that do not involve infection.

Neutralizing anti-MCP-1 antibodies have been used to document the pathogenetic role of MCP-1 in several renal disorders. In a rat model of glomerulonephritis induced by anti-glomerular basement membrane antibodies, anti-MCP-1 antibodies decreased early monocyte infiltration and proteinuria [24, 25]. In another model, crescentic glomerulonephritis can be induced in the rat by "nephrotoxic" sera. In this case, too, anti-MCP-1 antibodies reduced macrophage accumulation in glomeruli and reduced crescent formation and proteinuria [26]. Similar results were observed in a mouse model of crescentic glomerulonephritis [27]. Finally, anti-MCP-1 antibody administration decreased the severity of glomerulonephritis in a rat model induced by anti-thymocyte globulin [28]. Taken together, these diverse models indicate that MCP-1 expression may be a critical component of the final common pathway that results in glomerular injury and proteinuria.

Murine models of asthma have been developed in which airway inflammation and bronchial hyperresponsiveness can be induced by intranasal administration of an allergen in sensitized animals. Neutralization of MCP-1 in these models leads to an impressive reduction both in inflammation and hyperresponsiveness [29].

Small molecule MCP-1 antagonists are not widely available, but a potent peptide inhibitor has been described. Removal of amino acids 2–8 results in a variant, termed 7ND, that inhibits wild type MCP-1 activity *in vitro* with an IC_{50} that occurs at a molar ratio of 75:1, or approximately 35 nM at physiological MCP-1 concentrations [8]. As noted above, its mechanism of action is still unclear and it may act as a dominant negative inhibitor or as a competitive inhibitor at the MCP-1 receptor. A similar N-terminally truncated variant in which amino acids 1–8 have been removed is denoted 9–76 [9]. This peptide can reduce the incidence and severity of autoimmune arthritis in MRL-lpr mice treated with complete Freund's adjuvant [30]. While this is an impressive demonstration of an MCP-1 inhibitor's ability to treat arthritis in the mouse, it does not directly prove that MCP-1 is responsible for arthritis. This inference would require a demonstration that MCP-1 9–76 is specific for MCP-1, and although this is likely to be true, it has not been rigorously demonstrated.

Perhaps the best way to demonstrate MCP-1's pathogenetic involvement in disease is through the use of genetics. Both $MCP-1^{-/-}$ and $CCR2^{-/-}$ animals have been tested in models of atherosclerosis. Disrupted $MCP-1$ alleles were placed in a low density lipoprotein receptor deficient background, and animals were fed high cholesterol diets [31]. Despite the fact that $MCP-1^{-/-}$ and $MCP-1^{+/+}$ mice had identical plasma cholesterol levels and lipoprotein profiles, the $MCP-1^{-/-}$ mice had 80% less lipid deposition in their aortas. Furthermore, this difference persisted during 25 weeks of hypercholesterolemia, indicating that the absence of plaques in MCP-1-deficient animals was not due to delayed development of disease. Mechanistically, fewer macrophages were found in the aortic walls of the MCP-1-deficient animals suggesting that in the absence of MCP-1, blood monocytes were not recruited into the aortic subendothelium where they would ordinarily become the foam cells of atherosclerotic plaques.

In similar experiments, disrupted $CCR2$ alleles were placed in an apoE-deficient background [32]. Again, despite having similar levels of total cholesterol and lipoproteins, the $CCR2^{-/-}$ mice had less lipid deposition in their aortas than $CCR2^{+/+}$ animals, although there was some disease advancement as the period of hypercholesterolemia continued. As in the $MCP-1^{-/-}$ mice, fewer macrophages were found in the aortic walls of $CCR2^{-/-}$ mice. Thus in two distinct models of atherosclerosis, the MCP-1/CCR2 axis has been found to be essential for disease development. In patients with refractory hypercholesterolemia, e.g. those with familial hypercholesterolemia or individuals resistant to statins, anti-MCP-1 or CCR2 therapy may reduce their risk of atherosclerosis.

Conclusion

While MCP-1's involvement in inflammatory disease had always made sense based on its *in vitro* properties, only recently have the tools been available to directly demonstrate MCP-1's pathogenetic role. The antibody, peptide inhibitor, and "knockout" data all point to unique roles for MCP-1 and CCR2 in a variety of abnormalities characterized by monocyte or lymphocyte recruitment. These observations validate MCP-1 and CCR2 as drug targets and suggest that antagonists directed against these molecules will be therapeutically beneficial.

Reference

1   Cochran BH, Reffel AC, Stiles CD (1983) Molecular cloning of gene sequences regulated by platelet-derived growth factor. *Cell* 33: 939–947
2   Rollins BJ, Morrison ED, Stiles CD (1988) Cloning and expression of JE, a gene

inducible by platelet-derived growth factor and whose product has cytokine-like properties. *Proc Natl Acad Sci USA* 85: 3738–3742

3   Valente AJ, Graves DT, Vialle-Valentin CE, Delgado R, Schwartz CJ (1988) Purification of a monocyte chemotactic factor secreted by nonhuman primate vascular cells in culture. *Biochem* 27: 4162–4168

4   Yoshimura T, Robinson EA, Tanaka S, Appella E, Kuratsu JI, Leonard EJ (1989) Purification and amino acid analysis of two human glioma-derived monocyte chemoattractants. *J Exp Med* 169: 1449–1459

5   Matsushima K, Larsen CG, DuBois GC, Oppenheim JJ (1989) Purification and characterization of a novel monocyte chemotactic and activating factor produced by a human myelomonocytic cell line. *J Exp Med* 169: 1485–1490

6   Charo IF, Myers SJ, Herman A, Franci C, Connolly AJ, Coughlin SR (1994) Molecular cloning and functional expression of two monocyte chemoattractant protein 1 receptors reveals alternative splicing of the carboxyl-terminal tails. *Proc Natl Acad Sci USA* 91: 2752–2756

7   Yen H, Penfold S, Zhang Y, Rollins BJ (1997) MCP-1-mediated chemotaxis requires activation of non-overlapping signal tranduction pathways. *J Leuk Biol* 61: 529–532

8   Zhang YJ, Rutledge BJ, Rollins BJ (1994) Structure/activity analysis of human monocyte chemoattractant protein-1 (MCP-1) by mutagenesis: identification of a mutated protein that inhibits MCP-1-mediated monocyte chemotaxis. *J Biol Chem* 269: 15918–15924

9   Gong JH, Clark-Lewis I (1995) Antagonists of monocyte chemoattractant protein 1 identified by modification of functionally critical NH2-terminal residues. *J Exp Med* 181: 631–640

10 Zhang Y, Rollins BJ (1995) A dominant negative inhibitor indicates that monocyte chemoattractant protein 1 functions as a dimer. *Mol Cell Biol* 15: 4851–4855

11 Zachariae COC, Anderson AO, Thompson HL, Appella E, Mantovani A, Oppenheim JJ, Matsushima K (1990) Properties of monocyte chemotactic and activating factor (MCAF) purified from a human fibrosarcoma cell line. *J Exp Med* 171: 2177–2182

12 Ernst CA, Zhang YJ, Hancock PR, Rutledge BJ, Corless CL, Rollins BJ (1994) Biochemical and biological characterization of murine MCP-1: Identification of two functional domains. *J Immunol* 152: 3541–3549

13 Rutledge BJ, Rayburn H, Rosenberg R, North RJ, Gladue RP, Corless CL, Rollins BJ (1995) High level monocyte chemoattractant protein-1 expression in transgenic mice increases their susceptibility to intracellular pathogens. *J Immunol* 155: 4838–4843

14 Fuentes ME, Durham SK, Swerdel MR, Lewin AC, Barton DS, Megill JR, Bravo R, Lira SA (1995) Controlled recruitment of monocytes/macrophages to specific organs through transgenic expression of MCP-1. *J Immunol* 155: 5769–5776

15 Nakamura K, Williams IR, Kupper TS (1995) Keratinocyte-derived monocyte chemoattractant protein 1 (MCP-1): analysis in a transgenic model demonstrates MCP-1 can recruit dendritic and Langerhans cells to skin. *J Invest Dermatol* 105: 635–643

16 Gunn MD, Nelken NA, Liao X, Williams LT (1997) Monocyte chemoattractant pro-

tein-1 is sufficient for the chemotaxis of monocytes and lymphocytes in transgenic mice but requires an additional stimulus for inflammatory activation. *J Immunol* 158: 376–383

17 Kolattukudy PE, Quach T, Bergese S, Breckenridge S, Hensley J, Altschuld R, Gordillo G, Klenotic S, Orosz C, Parker-Thornburg J (1998) Myocarditis induced by targeted expression of the MCP-1 gene in murine cardiac muscle. *Am J Pathol* 152: 101–111

18 Grewal IS, Rutledge BJ, Fiorillo JA, Gu L, Gladue RP, Flavell RA, Rollins BJ (1997) Transgenic monocyte chemoattractant protein-1 (MCP-1) in pancreatic islets produces monocyte-rich insulitis without diabetes: abrogation by a second transgene expressing systemic MCP-1. *J Immunol* 159: 401–408

19 Lu B, Rutledge BJ, Gu L, Fiorillo J, Lukacs NW, Kunkel SL, North R, Gerard C, Rollins BJ (1998) Abnormalities in monocyte recruitment and cytokine expression in monocyte chemoattractant protein 1-deficient mice. *J Exp Med* 187: 601–608

20 Boring L, Gosling J, Chensue SW, Kunkel SL, Farese RVJ, Broxmeyer HE, Charo IF (1997) Impaired monocyte migration and reduced type 1 (Th1) cytokine responses in C-C chemokine receptor 2 knockout mice. *J Clin Invest* 100: 2552–2561

21 Kurihara T, Warr G, Loy J, Bravo R (1997) Defects in macrophage recruitment and host defense in mice lacking the CCR2 chemokine receptor. *J Exp Med* 186: 1757–1762

22 Kuziel WA, Morgan SJ, Dawson TC, Griffin S, Smithies O, Ley K, Maeda N (1997) Severe reduction in leukocyte adhesion and monocyte extravasation in mice deficient in CC chemokine receptor 2. *Proc Natl Acad Sci USA* 94: 12053–12058

23 Karpus WJ, Lukacs NW, Kennedy KJ, Smith WS, Hurst SD, Barrett TA (1997) Differential CC chemokine-induced enhancement of T helper cell cytokine production. *J Immunol* 158: 4129–4136

24 Fujinaka H, Yamamoto T, Takeya M, Feng L, Kawasaki K, Yaoita E, Kondo D, Wilson CB, Uchiyama M, Kihara I (1997) Suppression of anti-glomerular basement membrane nephritis by administration of anti-monocyte chemoattractant protein-1 antibody in WKY rats. *J Am Soc Nephrol* 8: 1174–1178

25 Tang WW, Qi M, Warren JS (1996) Monocyte chemoattractant protein 1 mediates glomerular macrophage infiltration in anti-GBM Ab GN. *Kidney Intl* 50: 665–671

26 Wada T, Yokoyama H, Furuichi K, Kobayashi KI, Harada K, Naruto M, Su SB, Akiyama M, Mukaida N, Matsushima K (1996) Intervention of crescentic glomerulonephritis by antibodies to monocyte chemotactic and activating factor (MCAF/MCP-1). *FASEB J* 10: 1418–1425

27 Lloyd CM, Minto AW, Dorf ME, Proudfoot A, Wells TN, Salant DJ, Gutierrez-Ramos JC (1997) RANTES and monocyte chemoattractant protein-1 (MCP-1) play an important role in the inflammatory phase of crescentic nephritis, but only MCP-1 is involved in crescent formation and interstitial fibrosis. *J Exp Med* 185: 1371–1380

28 Wenzel U, Schneider A, Valente AJ, Abboud HE, Thaiss F, Helmchen UM, Stahl RA (1997) Monocyte chemoattractant protein-1 mediates monocyte/macrophage influx in anti-thymocyte antibody-induced glomerulonephritis. *Kidney Intl* 51: 770–776

29 Gonzalo JA, Lloyd CM, Wen D, Albar JP, Wells TN, Proudfoot A, Martinez AC, Dorf

M, Bjerke T, Coyle AJ, Gutierrez-Ramos JC (1998) The coordinated action of CC chemokines in the lung orchestrates allergic inflammation and airway hyperresponsiveness. *J Exp Med* 188: 157–167

30   Gong JH, Ratkay LG, Waterfield JD, Clark-Lewis I (1997) An antagonist of monocyte chemoattractant protein 1 (MCP-1) inhibits arthritis in the MRL-lpr mouse model. *J Exp Med* 186: 131–137

31   Gu L, Okada Y, Clinton SK, Gerard C, Sukhova GK, Libby P, Rollins BJ (1998) Absence of monocyte chemoattractant protein-1 reduces atherosclerosis in low density lipoprotein receptor-deficient mice. *Mol Cell* 2: 275–281

32   Boring L, Gosling J, Cleary M, Charo IF (1998) Decreased lesion formation in CCR2$^{-/-}$ mice reveals a role for chemokines in the initiation of atherosclerosis. *Nature* 394: 894–897

The role of chemokines in allergic diseases of the airways

Lisa A. Beck, Cristiana Stellato, Syed Shahabuddin, Renate Nickel and Robert P. Schleimer

Johns Hopkins University School of Medicine, Asthma and Allergy Center, 5501 Hopkins Bayview Circle, Baltimore, MD 21224, USA

Introduction

Allergic diseases of the airways such as asthma, rhinitis and sinusitis, are characterized by numerous pathological changes, including excess mucous secretion, hypertrophy of mucous glands and smooth muscle, edema of the tissue, epithelial denudation and thickening of basement membrane. With respect to chemokine biology, however, the most relevant feature is the intense infiltration of submucosal tissue with inflammatory cells, especially eosinophils, lymphocytes, monocytes and basophils [1]. This pattern of cellular infiltration is reproduced by experimental antigen challenge with intranasal or inhaled allergens in allergic subjects. There are many points in the cascade of cellular recruitment at which chemokines could theoretically play a role. For example, selected chemokines can alter bone marrow colony formation and/or transit of inflammatory cells from bone marrow to peripheral circulation [2]. A role is also clearly established for chemokines in adhesion and transendothelial migration of various leukocytes at sites of inflammation [3]. Chemokines are implicated in the localization of eosinophils and other cells to the mucosal region immediately adjacent to the epithelium as well as in the lumen of the airways [4, 5]. Chemokines have also been implicated as regulators of angiogenesis, T-cell differentiation, and other responses which may play a role in allergic disease [6]. The focus of this review is the potential role of eosinophil-active chemokines such as eotaxin, RANTES and MCP-4 in allergic diseases, with particular emphasis on the production of these chemokines by airway epithelial cells [7]. Another theme that runs through this review is the existence of differences in chemokine biology between individuals of African descent and Caucasians. These differentiating characteristics may be notable in so far as asthma mortality in the U.S. is disproportionately large in African-Americans [8].

Inflammatory Processes: Molecular Mechanisms and Therapeutic Opportunities, edited by L. Gordon Letts and Douglas W. Morgan
© 2000 Birkhäuser Verlag Basel/Switzerland

Genetic studies of asthma

Genome-wide screens and candidate gene approaches in populations of different ethnicities have shown evidence for linkage to a growing number of chromosomal regions of phenotypes associated with asthma (i.e. symptoms, IgE responses, bronchial hyperresponsiveness, etc.) [9–11]. In a genome-wide screen performed by the Collaborative Study for the Genetics of Asthma (CSGA), evidence was obtained for linkage of asthma to chromosome 17, the chromosome which contains one of the main C-C chemokine clusters, including MCPs, RANTES, eotaxin, etc. [9, 12, 13]. Interestingly, multipoint analysis on chromosome 17 showed significant results only for African-American and not Caucasian-American sibpairs. These findings led to further analysis of the RANTES gene by SSCP and DNA sequencing, which revealed an alternative allele to the reported wild-type of the RANTES promoter [14]. In this second allele, a point mutation results in the formation of a new consensus element for the GATA transcription factor family. Interestingly, this alternative allele is found much more frequently in populations of African descent than Caucasian subjects, with the homozygous form appearing ≤1% in the latter, and between 15 and 25% in the former. Preliminary functional studies suggest a higher constitutive transcriptional activity of the mutant promoter allele than the wild type in human cell lines expressing both RANTES and GATA-binding proteins. While this allele has not been associated with asthma in any of the tested populations, it is notable that RANTES may have important roles in diseases other than allergic diseases, including AIDS, renal diseases, etc. [15–17]. Further studies are necessary to determine whether the biological relevance of this promoter is cell type-dependent. For example, differential expression of GATA-3 has been shown in Th2 vs Th1 cells [18, 19]. The relevance of GATA proteins to RANTES expression in other cells such as fibroblasts, endothelial cells and epithelial cells is presently unknown.

Chemokines and eosinophil migration

It has long been hypothesized that the ability of chemokines to induce specific recruitment of eosinophils, and other cells involved in allergic reactions, may depend upon the occurrence of other important events. Both endothelial activation and eosinophil priming can quantitatively and qualitatively influence the eosinophil response to chemokines. This notion was initially based on *in vitro* studies showing that resting eosinophils do not actively traverse an unstimulated endothelial monolayer [20]. When the endothelial cells are activated by IL-1 or TNF, transendothelial migration of eosinophils increases three- to five-fold [20]. If the eosinophils are first cultured with a priming cytokine, such as IL-5, for two days, the transendothelial migration increases about ten-fold [21]. While a chemokine alone, such as RANTES, is an effective inducer of eosinophil transendothelial migration *in vitro*, when the eosinophils are first primed by exposure to a small amount of IL-5 or GM-CSF, the dose-response curve for RANTES in inducing eosinophil transendothelial migration is shifted to the left as well as upward, such that the maximal response is considerably greater [22]. Subsequent studies in animal models have established the importance of exposure to priming cytokines in producing chemokine-induced cell recruitment *in vivo* [23, 24]. In humans, injection of RANTES intracutaneously induces a profound eosinophil infiltration [25]. The kinetics of this response are dramatically influenced by the allergic status of the subject being challenged. Non-allergic individuals displayed a very slow response, with eosinophil recruitment only being apparent after 24 h, whereas allergic individuals showed eosinophil recruitment within 30 min [25].

We noted subsequently that two of the individuals that showed the most rapid and extensive eosinophil recruitment in response to RANTES injection are African-Americans and their erythrocytes are negative for the Duffy antigen, a 7TM receptor found on endothelial cells and erythrocytes. This receptor promiscuously binds chemokines and has been proposed to be a sink which quenches chemokine actions in the periphery [26]. While erythrocytes of Caucasians are primarily Duffy positive, virtually all African's erythrocytes are Duffy negative. Approximately 30% of African-American's erythrocytes are Duffy positive as a result of Caucasian admixture (reviewed in Hadley [27]). The absence of erythrocyte Duffy in all Africans provides an evolutionary advantage where malarial parasites are endemic, since Duffy-negative erythrocytes are resistant to infection by plasmodium vivax [28]. We are attempting to determine whether the status of Duffy expression on erythrocytes influences the response to injected chemokines or allergen.

Probably the most important explanation of the rapid response to RANTES injection in allergic individuals relates to the status of priming of circulating eosinophils. In these studies allergic and normal subjects were matched to have equivalent peripheral blood eosinophil counts [25]. Therefore, the dramatic increase in the rate of the response may relate to the increased adhesive and migratory responses of primed eosinophils. To better study priming, we have attempted to identify markers of eosinophil priming by screening the antibodies from the 5th International Workshop on Human Leukocyte Antigens. These studies revealed that CD44 and CD69 are significantly increased by priming of human eosinophils *in vitro* or *in vivo* [29]. Interestingly, when we assayed CD44 expression in a group of subjects, we found substantially higher levels in allergics than in normals. Furthermore, we found a correlation between CD44 expression and expression of CCR3, the receptor mediating eosinophil chemotaxis in response to several CC chemokines [30]. This finding indicates that CCR3 is more highly expressed in allergic subjects than normals, and that an increase in CCR3 may also result from priming of eosinophils. While *in vitro* studies indicate that cytokines such as IL-5 induce CD44 expression, such studies have failed to find induction of CCR3 expression. The mechanisms by which CCR3 is increased on the eosinophil surface of allergic subjects are still unknown.

CCR3 and eosinophil recruitment

In vitro studies showed that the response of eosinophils to C-C chemokines such as eotaxin, MCP-4 and RANTES is completely blocked by a specific anti-CCR3 antibody (developed by Drs. Paul Ponath and Charles Mackay at LeukoSite) [31]. Furthermore, the binding of radiolabeled eotaxin to peripheral blood eosinophils is inhibited by a variety of chemokines with a pattern almost identical to the pattern of binding to CCR3 transfectants [32]. In collaboration with Drs. Mary Brawner and Mary Barnett at SmithKline Beecham, we have screened human eosinophils for approximately 20 known and orphan chemokine receptors. Thus far, only CCR1 and CCR3 mRNA were detected in these cells (S. Shahabuddin et al., unpublished observations). Taken together, these studies support the contention that CCR3 is the primary receptor mediating chemokine-induced eosinophil chemotaxis. *In vivo* challenge of humans with MIP-1α, a CCR1 agonist, induced quite a modest influx of eosinophils, which was not greater in allergics than normals, and which represented approximately 3% of the total infiltrate (roughly the percentage of eosinophils of total leukocytes found in the peripheral blood) [33]. Considering the rapid advances in this area of research, and the fact that several groups have recently found additional eosinophil-active chemokines it will not be surprising if eosinophil migration is later found to be induced by receptors other than CCR3 and CCR1.

The mechanism by which chemokines stimulate migration and transendothelial migration is under active investigation. Recent studies have demonstrated an increased tethering of eosinophils to VCAM-1 and other surfaces by exposure to eotaxin [34]. In addition, Tachimoto and Bochner have shown that CCR3 agonists can cause a de-adherence of β1 integrins in the context of an increased β2 integrin-mediated adhesion [35]. Thus, following initial tethering of eosinophils to a surface expressing selectins and VCAM-1, it is possible that chemokines assist in the transition of cells from a β1-mediated response to the β2-mediated response which mediates transendothelial migration and migration within the tissue.

CCR3 and stromal cells

Recent studies have shown that CCR3 expression occurs in sessile cell types such as endothelial cells and epithelial cells [36, 37]. This expression has been confirmed with Western and Northern blot analysis, and immunohistochemistry. Preliminary studies indicate functional activity of this receptor based on calcium flux. Given the potential importance of CCR3 in allergic cell recruitment, further studies are in order to determine whether CCR3 on epithelial cells regulates either chemokine expression or other epithelial cell functions.

Generation of CC chemokines in human airways

Numerous studies have addressed the question of whether eosinophil-active CC chemokines are generated in the airways of either diseased allergic subjects or following experimental antigen challenge in asymptomatic allergic individuals [38]. While there is substantial variability in the responses observed, the general consensus is that most of these chemokines are found at increased concentrations in either nasal or lung lavage fluids following either antigen challenge or in asthmatic or allergic individuals. In some but not all cases, levels correlated with the influx of eosinophils. We must now make efforts to discriminate among the eosinophil-active CC chemokines to identify which one(s) is the most important in driving the inflammatory response. Emerging data indicate that RANTES may be less important than eotaxin, eotaxin-2 or MCP-4. Another important question relates to the cellular sources of these chemokines. Early studies indicate that airway epithelium stains brightly for RANTES, eotaxin and MCP-4 in human nasal polyps [4, 39, 40]. Cultured airway epithelial cells are an extremely rich source of RANTES, MCP-4, eotaxin and other chemokines. Interestingly, stimulus specificity is observed. For example, TNFα is a rapid inducer of epithelial production of eotaxin and MCP-4, and slowly induces RANTES expression [41]. Expression of eotaxin and MCP-4 occurs at substantially lower concentrations of TNFα than expression of RANTES, suggesting that mild inflammatory responses in the airways may selectively induce eotaxin and MCP-4. Recent interesting studies indicate that IL-4 strongly potentiates TNFα-induced production of eotaxin but not RANTES by airway epithelial cells (Stellato et al., unpublished observations). This raises the possibility that Th2 cells, by virtue of producing IL-4, may differentially regulate epithelial chemokine expression.

Glucocorticoids and the regulation of chemokine mRNA stability

Glucocorticoids are probably the most effective and among the most widely used medications for treatment of airways allergic diseases. The expression of eosinophil-active CC chemokines by airway epithelial cells is inhibited by glucocorticoids to a greater or lesser extent, depending on the stimulus and the chemokine in question [42]. This regulation is partly at the transcriptional level, based on studies using reporter gene systems and transfection of glucocorticoid-treated airway epithelial cells (Stellato et al., unpublished observations). Studies on mRNA stability, however, indicate that glucocorticoids destabilize eotaxin mRNA without a similar effect on RANTES mRNA [41]. This observation suggested to us that the stability-conferring regions of the 3'untranslated region (UTR) may be involved in the steroid effect, since previous publications have shown that the 3'UTR of eotaxin mRNA contains AU-rich elements (ARE) while that of RANTES does not. We are presently testing this hypothesis using an elegant system developed by Dr. Ann-Bin Shyu [43]. Because of its potential role in regulation of eotaxin expression, a search for polymorphisms of the 3'UTR of eotaxin in human subjects has been made. This region is extremely polymorphic, whereas the flanking, non AU-rich regions appear to be conserved (Nickel et al., manuscript in preparation). Among the polymorphisms are point mutations in the ARE as well as variability in length of adjacent poly U stretches also known to be involved in mRNA stability [43]. Using primers flanking the ARE, six different length allelic forms have been observed in African-Americans and three different forms have been observed in Caucasian-Americans ranging from 219 to 224 base pairs in length. Interestingly, transmission disequilibrium tests showed evidence for linkage and association of these alleles to asthma and asthma-associated phenotypes in two populations of African descent [14]. Whether there is a functional relationship between these molecular variants and stability of eotaxin mRNA remains to be determined.

Conclusion and summary

While chemokines clearly play a role in allergic diseases, the extent and the nature of that role is still unclear. The demonstration that selective chemokines can reproduce aspects of allergic inflammation and the ability of blockers to inhibit allergic inflammation in animal systems, coupled with increased production in human disease and allergen challenge models all support this conclusion. The precise relevance of individual CC chemokines discussed in this brief review is still unknown. Presumably, differential expression among chemokines induced by various cytokines and differential regulation of their expression by glucocorticoids *in vitro* reflect differences in their underlying regulation *in vivo*. As we begin to piece together chemokine responses *in vitro*, these *in vivo* regulatory pathways may become more clear. Finally, it is apparent that strong ethnic variations exist in the chemokine ligand and receptor pathways. Differences between individuals of African and European descent exist in the expression of Duffy on erythrocytes [28], the presence of the Δ32 CCR5 mutant [44], the RANTES promoter mutation discussed above, and the polymorphisms of the eotaxin 3'UTR. Recently, ethnic differences have been found in the prevalence of polymorphisms in the high affinity IgE receptor encoding gene [45]. It appears likely that distinctly different pressures on the immune system of ethnic groups living in Africa and Europe have resulted in divergence at a number of levels in the chemokine network. Whether these differences explain the different susceptibility or mortality of asthma or other diseases is a question which is only beginning to be addressed.

References

1   Bousquet J, Chanez P, Lacoste JY, Barneon G, Ghavanian N, Enander I, Venge P, Ahlstedt, Simony-Lafontaine J, Godard P, Michel FB (1990) Eosinophilic inflammation in asthma. *New Engl J Med* 323: 1033–1039

2   Quackenbush EJ, Aguirre V, Wershil BK, Gutierrez-Ramos JC (1997) Eotaxin influences the development of embryonic hematopoietic progenitors in the mouse. *J Leuk Biol* 62: 661–666

3   Lukacs NW, Strieter RM, Kunkel SL (1997) In: BS Bochner (ed): Adhesion molecules in allergic disease. Marcel Dekker, New York, 375–392

4   Beck LA, Stellato C, Beall LD, Schall TJ, Leopold D, Bickel CA, Baroody F, Bochner BS, Schleimer RP (1996) Detection of the chemokine RANTES and endothelial adhesion molecules in nasal polyps. *J Allergy Clin Immunol* 98: 766–780

5   Gonzalo J-A, Lloyd CM, Kremer L, Finger E, Martinez-A C, Siegelman MH, Cybulsky M, Gutierrez-Ramos J-C (1996) Eosinophil recruitment to the lung in a murine model of allergic inflammation The role of T cells, chemokines, and adhesion receptors. *J Clin Invest* 98: 2332–2345

6   Luster AD (1998) Chemokines-chemotactic cytokines that mediate inflammation. *New Engl J Med* 338: 436–445, 1998

7   Schwiebert LM, Stellato C, Schleimer RP (1996) The epithelium as a target of glucocorticoid action in the treatment of asthma. *Am J Respir Crit Care Med* 154: S16–S20

8   Cunningham J, Dockery DW, Speizer FE (1996) Race, asthma, and persistent wheeze in philadelphia schoolchildren. *J Public Health* 86: 1406–1409

9   The Collaborative Study on the Genetics of Asthma (1997) A genome-wide search for asthma susceptibility loci in ethnically diverse populations. *Nature Genet* 15: 389–392

10   Daniels SE, Bhattacharrya S, James A, Leaves NI, Young A, Hill MR, Faux JA, Ryan GF, leSouef PN, Lathrop GM, Musk AW, Cookson WOCM (1996) A genome wide search for quantitative trait loci underlying asthma. *Nature* 383: 247–250

11   Holgate ST (1997) Asthma genetics: waiting to exhale. *Nature Genet* 15: 227–229

12   Naruse K, Ueno M, Satoh T, Nomiyama H, Tei H, Takeda M, Ledbetter DH, VanCoillie E, Opdenakker G, Gunge B, Sakaki Y, Iio M, Miura R (1986) A YAC contig of the human CC chemokine genes clustered on chromosome 17q112. *Genomics* 34: 236–240

13   Garcia-Zepeda EA, Rothenberg ME, Weremowicz S, Sarafi MN, Morton CC, Luster AD (1997) Genomic organization, complete sequence, and chromosomal location of the gene for human eotaxin (SCYA11), and eosinophil-specific CC chemokine. *Genomics* 41: 471–476

14   Nickel R, Barnes KC, Sengler CA, Casolaro V, Friedhoff LR, Weber P, Naidu RP, Cora-

ballo L, Ehrlich E, Plitt J, Schleimer RP, CSGA T, Huang SK, Beaty T (1999) Evidence for linkage of chemokine polymorphisms to asthma in populations of african descent. *J Allergy Clin Immunol; in press*

15 Cocchi F, DeVico AL, Garzino-Demo A, Arya SK, Gallo RC, Lusso P (1995) Identification of RANTES, MIP-1 alpha, and MIP-1 beta as the major HIV-suppressive factors produced by CD8[+] T cells. *Science* 270: 1811–1815

16 Heeger P, Wolf G, Meyers C, Sun MJ, O'Farrell SC, Krensky AM, Neilson EG (1992) Isolation and characterization of cDNA from renal tubular epithelium encoding murine RANTES. *Kidney Intl* 41: 220–225

17 Pattison J, Nelson PJ, Huie P, von Leuttichau I, Farshid G, Sibley RK, Krensky AM (1994) RANTES chemokine expression in cell-mediated transplant rejection of the kidney. *Lancet* 343: 209–211

18 Zhang D-H, Cohn L, Ray P, Bottomly K (1997) A ray transcription factor GATA-3 is differentially expressed in murine Th1 and Th2 cells and controls Th2-specific expression of the interleukin-5 gene. *J Biol Chem* 272: 21597–21603

19 Zheng WP, Flavell A (1997) The transcription factor GATA-3 is necessary and sufficient fro the Th2 cytokine gene expression in CD4 T cells. *Cell* 89: 587–596

20 Ebisawa M, Bochner BS, Georas SN, Schleimer RP (1992) Eosinophil transendothelial migration induced by cytokines. I. Role of endothelial and eosinophil adhesion molecules in IL-1β-induced transendothelial migration. *J Immunol* 149: 4021–4028

21 Ebisawa M, Liu MC, Yamada T, Kato M, Lichtenstein LM, Bochner BS, Schleimer RP (1994) Eosinophil transendothelial migration induced by cytokines. II. The potentiation of eosinophil transendothelial migration by eosinophil-active cytokines. *J Immunol* 152: 4590–4597

22 Ebisawa M, Yamada T, Bickel C, Klunk D, Schleimer RP (1994) Eosinophil transendothelial migration induced by cytokines. III. Effect of the chemokine RANTES. *J Immunol* 153: 2153–2160

23 Meurer R, Van Riper G, Feeney W, Cunningham P, Hora D Jr, Springer MS, MacIntyre DE, Rosen H (1993) Formation of eosinophilic and monocytic intradermal inflammatory sites in the dog by injection of human RANTES but not human monocyte chemoattractant protein 1, human macrophage inflammatory protein 1α, or human interleukin 8. *J Exp Med* 178: 1913–1921

24 Collins PD, Marleau S, Griffiths-Johnson DA, Jose PJ, Williams TJ (1995) Cooperation between interleukin-5 and the chemokine eotaxin to induce eosinophil accumulation *in vivo*. *J Exp Med* 182: 1169–1174

25 Beck LA, Dalke S, Leiferman KM, Bickel CA, Hamilton R, Rosen H, Bochner BS, Schleimer RP (1997) Cutaneous injection of RANTES causes eosinophil recruitment: Comparison of nonallergic and allergic subjects. *J Immunol* 159: 2962–2972

26 Horuk R, Martin A, Hesselgesser J, Hadley T, Lu Z-H, Wang Z-X, Peiper SC (1996) The Duffy antigen receptor for chemokines: structural analysis and expression in the brain. *J Leuk Biol* 59: 29–38

27 Hadley TJ, Peiper SC (1997) From malaria to chemokine receptor: The emerging physiologic role of the Duffy blood group antigen. *Blood* 89: 3077–3091

28 Miller LH, Mason SJ, Clyde DF, McGinnis MH (1976) The resistance factor to *Plasmodium vivax* in blacks. The Duffy-blood-group genotype, FyFy. *N Engl J Med* 295: 302–304

29 Matsumoto K, Appiah-Pippim J, Schleimer RP, Bickel C, Beck LA, Bochner BS (1998) CD44 and CD69 represent different types of cell-surface activation markers for human eosinophils. *Am J Respir Cell Mol Biol* 18: 860–866

30 Beck LA, Brummet ME, Seminario M-C, Saini SS, Ponath PD, Bochner BS, Schleimer RP (1999) Surface expression of the chemokine receptor CCR3 on human eosinophils correlates with the activation marker CD44. *J Allergy Clin Immunol; in press*

31 Heath, H, S Qin, P Rao, L Wu, G LaRosa, N Kassam, PD Ponath, CR Mackay Chemokine receptor usage by human eosinophils. *J Clin Invest* 99: 178–184, 1997

32 Ponath PD, Qin S, Post TW, Wang J, Wu L, Gerard NP, Neuman W, Gerard C, Mackay CR (1996) Molecular cloning and characterization of a human eotaxin receptor expressed selectively on eosinophils *J Exp Med* 183: 2437–2448

33 Lee SC, Brummet ME, Woodworth T, Leiferman KM, Gilman S, Gladue R, Schleimer RP, Beck LA (1998) Cutaneous injection of human subjects with macrophage inflammatory protein-1α (MIP-1α) causes significant leukocyte recruitment. *J Allergy Clin Immunol* 101: A821

34 Kitayama J, Carr MW, Roth SJ, Buccola J, Springer TA (1977) Contrasting responses to multiple chemotactic stimuli in transenodthelial migration. *J Immunol* 158: 2340–2349

35 Bochner BS, Sterbinsky SA, Tachimoto H (1999) CCR3-active chemokines rapidly inhibit human eosinophil adhesion to VCAM-1 *in vitro*. *J Allergy Clin Immunol; in press*

36 Sholl L, Brummet M, Stellato C, Seminario M-C, Plitt J, Ponath P, Bochner BS, Schleimer RP, Beck LA (1998) Detection of the chemokine receptor CCR3 on endothelial cells. *FASEB J* 12: A590

37 Stellato C, Brummet ME, Bickel CA, Ponath PD, Liu MC, Schleimer RP, Beck LA (1999) Characterization of CCR3 expression on human airway epithelial cells. *J Allergy Clin Immunol; in press*

38 Baggiolini M, Dewald B, Moser B (1997) Human chemokines: An update. *Annu Rev Immunol* 15: 675–705

39 Lamkhioued B, Renzi PM, Abi-Younes S, Garcia-Zepada EA, Allakhvberdi Z, Ghaffar O, Rothenberg MD, Luster AD, Hamid Q (1997) Increased expression of eotaxin in bronchoalveolar lavage and airways of asthmatic contributes to the chemotaxis of eosinophils to the site of inflammation. *J Immunol* 159: 4593–4601

40 Miotto D, Lamkhioued B, Taha R, Renzi P, Ghaffar O, Garcia-Zepeda E, Luster A, Hamid Q (1997) MCP-4 expression in asthmatic lungs. *Am J Respir Crit Care Med* 155: A817

41 Stellato C, Plitt JR, Bickel CA, White J, Schleimer RP (1998) Differential regulation of

epithelial-derived C-C chemokines by cytokines and budesonide. *J Allergy Clin Immunol* 101: S230

42 Stellato C, Schleimer RP (1999) In: M Rothenberg (ed) *Chemokines in allergic diseases.* Marcel Dekker, Inc, New York

43 Xu N, Chen C-YA, Shyu A-B (1997) Modulation of the fate of cytoplasmic mRNA by AU-rich elements: Key sequence features controlling mRNA deadenylation and decay. *Mol Cell Biol* 17: 4611–4621

44 Samson M, Libert F, Doranz BJ, Rucker J, Liesngard C, Farber C-M, Saragosti S, Lapoumeroulie C, Cognaux J, Forceille C et al (1996) Resistance to HIV-1 infection in caucasian individuals bearing mutant alleles of the CCR-5 chemokine receptor gene. *Nature* 382: 722–725

45 Green SL, Gaillard MC, Song E, Dewar JB, Halkas A (1998) Polymorphisms of the beta chain of the high-affinity immunoglobulin E receptor in South African black and white asthmatic and nonasthmatic individuals. *Am J Respir Crit Care Med* 158: 1487–14928

Inflammation Research Association
Ninth International Conference, November 1–5, 1998

Summaries of workshops and poster discussions

Coordinators:　　*James Winkler (SmithKline Beecham)*
　　　　　　　　　　Ken Tramposch (Bristol-Myers Squibb)

Targets in rheumatoid and osteoarthritis

Chairpersons: Willam Williams (SmithKline Beecham)
Elizabeth Arner (DuPont)

The workshop on "Targets in rheumatoid and osteoarthritis" focused primarily on two aspects of these diseases: matrix degradation and inflammation. The first three presentations were related to matrix degradation and focused primarily on either degradative cytokines or proteases which serve as targets for the development of disease modifying anti-arthritic drugs.

The first presentation by Dr. Leo Joosten (University Hospital Nijmegen, The Netherlands) addressed the importance of IL-1α and β versus TNFα as mediators of inflammation and cartilage degradation. Using a collagen-induced arthritis model in mice, they dosed from the onset of the disease at day 28 through day 36 with either sTNFα binding protein or with IL-1α and β antibodies. Although they found that both treatments with the sTNFα binding protein and with the combination of IL-1α and β antibodies inhibited inflammation, only treatment with the IL-1 antibodies inhibited cartilage and bone erosions; sTNFα binding protein was ineffective. In addition, these researchers found that serum cartilage oligomeric matrix protein (COMP) levels in this collagen induced arthritis model showed a significant (r^2 = 0.94) positive correlation with disease severity. Serum COMP levels were decreased by treatment with IL-1α and β antibodies, but not by treatment with sTNFα binding protein. These studies demonstrate that while both inflammation and matrix degradation are involved in arthritis, the matrix loss is independent of inflammation. This finding has implications for the development of treatments for rheumatoid arthritis. Any potential anti-arthritic drugs must be evaluated for both the ability to block inflammation and for the ability to prevent matrix degradation; it cannot be assumed a drug which blocks inflammation will also be efficacious in preventing cartilage loss.

Studies exploring the complex regulation of PGE_2 and stromelysin (MMP-3) production in human osteoarthritic cartilage by nitric oxide (NO) were presented by Dr. Ashok Amin (New York University, New York, NY). He demonstrated that human osteoarthritic cartilage spontaneously releases PGE_2, NO, and MMP-3 in culture. Inhibitors of NO production resulted in increased MMP-3 production and COX-2-mediated PGE_2 production, suggesting that NO inhibits this up-regulation

Inflammatory Processes: Molecular Mechanisms and Therapeutic Opportunities, edited by L. Gordon Letts and Douglas W. Morgan
© 2000 Birkhäuser Verlag Basel/Switzerland

of PGE_2. Addition of NO decreased NO, MMP-3 and PGE_2 production whereas addition of PGE_2 had no effect on NO production, but resulted in increased PGE_2 and MMP-3 production. Although the mechanism and pathways for this regulation is unclear, it suggests a complex control mechanism for the production of these mediators in human osteoarthritis.

The second presentation by Dr. Joosten for Dr. Lubberts (University Hospital Nijmegen, The Netherlands) examined the effect of adenoviral vector-mediated expression of IL-4 locally in mouse knee joints on collagen induced arthritis. Intra-articular injection of IL-4 expressing adenovirus vector prior to the onset of arthritis resulted in more severe inflammation in the knee joint. In contrast, IL-4 resulted in prevention of chondrocyte cell death and an increased synthesis of cartilage proteolgycan as monitored by ^{35}S-sulfate uptake compared with arthritic controls. In addition, IL-4 expression resulted in prevention of bone erosion and resulted in a down-regulation of expression of IL-1β, TNFα and MMP-3. The authors suggest that transfection and over-expression of IL-4 may provide a therapeutic approach for the treatment of arthritic diseases.

This presentation together with the first presentation of the session demonstrates that while both inflammation and matrix degradation are involved in arthritis, the matrix loss is independent of inflammation. This finding has implications for the development of treatments for rheumatoid arthritis. Any potential anti-arthritic drugs must be evaluated for both the ability to block inflammation and for the ability to prevent matrix degradation; it cannot be assumed a drug which blocks inflammation will also be efficacious in preventing cartilage loss.

The next three talks were involved with the inflammatory aspects of arthritis. Dr. van den Berg presented for Dr. Van de Loo on the distinct roles of interleukin-6 (IL-6) and nitric oxide (NO) in antigen-induced gonarthritis in mice. They used IL-6$^{-/-}$ and inducible nitric-oxide synthase (NOS2)$^{-/-}$ mice to explore effects on inflammation and cartilage pathology. Both types of knockout mice had relatively well preserved immune responses to methylated BSA (mBSA), although the IL-6$^{-/-}$ mice had a somewhat diminished antibody response. Upon instillation of mBSA into the mouse knee joints, both strains developed early inflammatory responses (day 1), but this resolved much more rapidly in the IL-6$^{-/-}$ mice. In addition, the IL-6$^{-/-}$ mice had much better preservation of cartilage with very little evidence of proteoglycan degradation. Late in the process (day 14), all of the IL-6$^{-/-}$ mice (13/13) had peaking at day 7, while clenoliximab was non-depleting. In the oxazalone induced contact sensitivity model, both mAbs administered prior to sensitization significantly inhibited the ear resolution of the arthritis, while the NOS2$^{-/-}$ mice had resolution in 17/30, compared with 4/32 controls. Somewhat different results were seen in immune complex-induced arthritis where the IL-6$^{-/-}$ were not protected, but the NOS2$^{-/-}$ mice were. Questions from the audience brought out the fact that fibroblast proliferation was diminished in the IL-6$^{-/-}$ mice. The potential for other NOS isoforms to compensate for the lack of NOS2 was raised, and Dr. van den Berg pointed out that NO and nitro-tyrosine were reduced in the NOS2$^{-/-}$ mice to 5–10% of control values.

The talk by Manjula Reddy et al. focussed on the use of mice that expressed the human CD4 gene in the absence of murine CD4 expression (murine CD4$^{-/-}$ human CD4$^+$ mice). They analyzed the effects of two human anti-CD4 monoclonal antibodies which are being investigated for the treatment of rheumatoid arthritis: keliximab (IgG1) and clenoliximab (IgG4 mutated to lack Fc receptor binding) in these mice. They showed that keliximab depleted CD4$^+$ T cells by up to 60%, swelling response as well as levels of IL-4 and interferon γ. If administered following sensitization, neither mAb was inhibitory. This indicates that CD4$^+$ T-cell depletion is not needed for inhibition of the afferent phase of contact sensitivity. Effects on Th-1 *versus* Th-2 cells were inquired about, but those studies have not been performed as yet.

The final talk by S. Shortkroff et al. investigated the use of magnetic resonance imaging (MRI) in evaluating steroid treatment *versus* radiation synovectomy in the antigen-induced arthritis (AIA) model in rabbits. Radiation synovectomy utilized intraarticular ^{90}Y-hydroxyapatite, and typically produces an acute inflammatory response due to the radiation damage, so a third group received radiation synovectomy plus intra-articular corticosteroids. The histologic evaluation and knee diameters, as expected, showed marked inflammation in the control and radiation synovectomy groups, and this was reduced in both groups receiving corticosteroids. The MRI studies showed marked enhancement with gadolinium-DTPA contrast, indicative of vascular permeability, and this was ameliorated at the earliest timepoint post contrast injection in both of the steroid-treated groups (correlating with the clinical and histologic evaluation). This indicates the utility of MRI in quantifying inflammation and vascular permeability in synovitis.

Overall, the portion of the session on inflammation was characterized by insights ranging from mediators to measurements. All came away with important new information about the role of specific cytokines, cell types, and outcome parameters which should be of considerable utility in the discovery and development of novel pharmacophores.

Signal transduction and regulation of gene expression

Chairpersons: Lawrence Wennogle (Novartis)
Nancy Cusack (Pfizer)

The race to develop drugs to pro-inflammatory mediators took an exciting leap forward during the IRA annual meeting in Hershey, Pennsylvania. The excitement was evident during the workshop "Signal transduction and regulation of gene expression" organized by N. Cusack, P. Changelian, and L. Wennogle. One highlight was the presentation of highly specific inhibitors of p38 kinase. In addition, powerful biotechnology tools were discussed which are being applied to reveal novel insights into intracellular signal transduction pathways.

Pharmacology of p38 and JNK pathways

Three of the talks discussed new developments in the p38 MAPK-regulated signaling events, which underscores the high level of interest in this molecule as a target for anti-inflammatory drugs. Melanie Allen (Pfizer) presented work on p38α knockout embryonic stem cells (ESC). Although p38α knockout mice do not survive to term, p38$\alpha^{-/-}$ ESC were isolated by neomycin selection. Wild-type ESC phosphorylate p38α and MAPKAP Kinase-2 in response to stress. In the knockout p38$\alpha^{-/-}$ cells, sodium arsenite-induced MAPKAP Kinase-2 phosphorylation was evident (and SB-203580-suppressible), but much reduced from the level seen in wild-type ESC and this difference could be attributed to p38. Recent data (Ben-Levy et al. (1988) *Current Biology* 8: 1049–1057) demonstrates that phosphorylation of MAP-KAP Kinase-2 is necessary for cytosolic localization of p38, which resides in a nuclear complex with unphosphorylated MAPKAP Kinase prior to activation. Loss of p38 in knockout cells should have implications for MAPKAP Kinase-2 localization. Further work with these knockout cells will clarify the roles of the different p38 isoforms in development and in inflammatory responses.

In a remarkable demonstration of the power of medicinal chemistry, Barry Burnette (Monsanto) presented highly specific inhibitors of the MAPK family with 100-fold selectivity for α over β and 1000-fold specificity for p38 over JNK isoforms. Although the MAP kinase family is highly conserved, particularly in the ATP binding site, it is known that single amino acid substitutions render these kinases either

Inflammatory Processes: Molecular Mechanisms and Therapeutic Opportunities, edited by L. Gordon Letts and Douglas W. Morgan

Table 1 - Kinase selectivity analysis (IC$_{50}$, μM)

Compound	p38α	p38β	p38γ/δ	JNK1	JNK2	JNK3	ERK2
SB-203580	0.22	0.9	>100	>200	5.7	20	>100
SC-335	0.011	0.15	>100	8.3	0.22	0.83	>100
SC-178	0.001	0.008	>100	7.7	0.33	3.2	>100
SC-889	0.045	2.9	>100	>200	66	>200	>100
SC-906	0.07	5.7	>100	>200	112	>200	>100

susceptible or insensitive to inhibitors such as SB203580. Burnette showed that U937 cells did not contain detectable levels of p38β, γ or δ. When these cells were stimulated with LPS, p38-specific inhibitors effectively blocked TNFα production and phosphorylation of MAPKAP kinase-2 with no apparent effects on the phosphorylation of c-Jun. One such inhibitor was active in the rat paw edema model. The inhibitors should be key reagents to test the attractive possibility that p38α isoform-specific inactivation may result in anti-inflammatory drugs with fewer side-effects (Tab. 1).

Lori Stillwell (Monsanto) utilized synovial fibroblasts to demonstrate the effectiveness of these p38 inhibitors in suppressing COX-2 induction by IL-1. Flow-cytometric analysis on permeabilized cells showed that p38 inhibitors blocked production of COX-2 protein and mRNA at the level of transcription while having no effect on COX-2 enzyme activity *in vitro*. The widely-used p38 inhibitor SB203580 inhibits TNFα and IL-1 production in human monocytes following LPS stimulation, reported to be at the level of protein translation. However, additional issues remain to be resolved such as the effects of different classes of p38 inhibitors on cyclooxygenase. A recent publication by Borsch-Haubold et al. (*JBC* 273 (1998): 28766–28722) reported that SB203580 exhibits inhibitory activity against purified COX-1, COX-2 and had an ability to scavenge free radicals. Further investigation is needed to clarify the activities directly attributable to p38 in these signaling pathways and the true specificities of various inhibitors of the MAPK family members *in vivo*.

Brydon Bennett (Signal Pharmaceuticals) discussed the effects of anti-inflammatory mediators on immune function. JURKAT cells respond to PMA, αCD3 and αCD28, or PMA and PHA with activation of IKK, JNK and IL-2 transcription. It was determined that inhibitors of either IKK or JNK, but not p38 or MEK-1, prevented the increase in transcription of IL-2. Further, dominant-negative IKK-2, JIP-1 or MEKK-1 also inhibited this response. Roger Davis has previously alluded to the fact that JNK-1 and JNK-2 knockout mice display significant immune dysfunction, with a loss of the ability to generate Th-1 responses. Double JNK knockouts are embryonic lethal, indicating some ability of one JNK isoform to compensate for the other. Although JNK inhibitors may be useful immunosuppressive agents, further investigation is needed, particularly to establish efficacy to inhibit MLR or Blast responses in peripheral blood leukocytes. A deficiency in IL-2 production is likely to be only one of a number of responses affected by the JNK signaling pathway since IL-2 knockout mice exhibit an immunocompetent phenotype. As with other MAPK cascades, the complexity of having a number of isoforms and multiple accessory molecules such as scaffolding proteins and upstream mediators will make this an active area of research for some time to come.

Model systems and technology

A model for analyzing LPS signaling pathways in insect cells was presented by William Cornwell (SmithKline Beecham). *Drosophila* S2 cells were transiently transfected with an LPS-responsive luciferase reporter construct (previously described) resulting in cells with significant responsiveness to LPS. Co-transfection with *dorsal* (rel homologue) resulted in increased LPS-responsiveness while co-transfection with either *relish* (NF-κB homologue) or *cactus* (IκB homologue) resulted in decreased responsiveness. In insect cells LPS signaling represents a conserved function of innate immunity and is known to be mediated through the Toll receptor. The question of relevance to mammalian systems arises, since these cells are not known to contain signaling pathways analogous to CD14. However, many mysteries remain in the mammalian signal transduction system and this insect model system has the advantage of powerful and simple genetics. A recent report by Yang et al. (*Nature* 395 (1998): 284–288) describes a significant role for Toll-like receptors in mammalian leukocytes which may provide some answers to the many remaining questions regarding LPS signaling.

Method for the identification of IL-1 responsive genes through differential display

G. Gorski (Thomas Jefferson University) presented a method for the identification of IL-1-responsive genes through differential display. Analysis of IL-1-stimulated synovial fibroblasts resulted in the identification of many genes known to be regulated by IL-1 including: c-Jun, MINOR, and TNFR II. A novel gene was upregulated six-fold with IL-1. Its function remains to be determined.

Natural products

The final presentation of this workshop focused on a natural product – cat's claw (*Uncaria tomentosa*) – utilized as a traditional treatment for gastrointestinal disorders by Peruvian natives. The bark of this plant is boiled to produce a tea, which is ingested to treat a variety of inflammatory disorders. Macrophage (RAW 264.7) and colonic epithelial cells (HT 29) were used to study the effects of cat's claw on cellular functions in response to peroxinitrite and LPS. Cells treated with the tea showed a marked reduction in apoptosis, nitrite formation, LPS-induced iNOS expression and NF-κB activation. Cat's claw was extremely effective in the inhibition of gastroenteropathy associated with indomethacin toxicity. The anti-oxidant and anti-inflammatory properties of this medicine are significant and the precedent for natural products, which are potent modulators of inflammatory and immune responses, is well appreciated. A group of alkaloids present in the extract were detailed, but the chemical or chemicals responsible for the therapeutic effects remain unidentified.

Mediators of inflammation and their enzymes

Chairpersons: *James Burke (Bristol-Myers Squibb)*
Floyd Chilton (Wake Forest University)

Francois Nantel (Merck Frosst) described work characterizing the regulation of cyclooxygenase-2 (COX-2) at the RNA, protein, and mediator (PGE_2) level in two similar models: the rat carrageenin-induced edema model and the rat carrageenin-induced hyperalgesia model. In both models, carrageenin induced both mRNA and protein levels of COX-2 along with PGE_2 levels. Interestingly, indomethacin completely abolished this induction in the edema model which suggests the existence of some positive feedback loop by which PGE_2 acts to regulate COX-2 expression. However, indomethacin had no effect on these levels in the model of hyperalgesia. Immunoreactivity towards COX-2 was only detected in the epidermis in the edema model where the hyperalgesia model also showed immunoreactivity in skeletal muscle and inflammatory cells. Differences in the amount of carrageenin administered in the two models along with an age difference in the rats used may explain these observations.

In a related presentation, Chistopher Smith of Searle showed that a COX-1 selective analog (SC-560) of celecoxib (Searle's COX-2 inhibitor in the clinic) was able to inhibit the carrageenin-induced PGE_2 levels in the rat paw to near baseline levels without affecting the edema or hyperalgesia. Conversely, celecoxib inhibited both PGE_2 levels and edema/hyperalgesia. This apparent paradox is most probably due to an inhibition of the baseline levels of PGE_2 (but not the induced levels) by SC-560. Indeed, dual COX-1/COX-2 inhibitors inhibited the carrageenin-induced PGE_2 levels to well below baseline levels. Interestingly, the COX-1 inhibitor (SC-560) showed no affect on carrageenin-induced PGE_2 levels in the cerebrospinal fluid while celecoxib showed marked reduction. This observation is consistent with the idea that COX-2-mediated PGE_2 production plays a critical neurological role in inflammation/hyperalgesia.

During a presentation on the relative levels of different isoforms of sPLA2 in inflammatory cells, Elizabeth Capper (SmithKline Beecham) showed by FACS analysis using specific antibodies that human monocytes contain the group V and not the group IIa isoform and that the enzyme remained intracellular even upon stimulation. Interestingly, rheumatoid synovial fibroblasts possessed both group IIa

Inflammatory Processes: Molecular Mechanisms and Therapeutic Opportunities, edited by L. Gordon Letts and Douglas W. Morgan

and V isoforms. This enzyme was shown in these cells to be secreted and associated with the cell surface upon stimulation.

In a related presentation, Floyd Chilton (Wake Forest University) provided evidence that in murine bone marrow-derived mast cells, sPLA2 induces arachidonate mobilization through its interaction with the sPLA2 receptor and not through sPLA2 enzymatic activity. This was evidenced by RT-PCR studies showing that the sPLA2 receptor is expressed in these cells and that the sPLA2 isotypes which selectively induced arachidonate release in these cells also had the capacity to bind to the receptors on mast cells. More convincingly, an agonist of the receptor, *p*-aminophenyl-a-D-mannopyranoside, selectively released AA from mast cells, mimicking the effect of sPLA2. Additional work demonstrated that sPLA2 binding to the receptor induced the activation and membrane translocation of the cytosolic phospholipase A2 (cPLA2), which appears to be the enzyme which actually catalyzes the release of arachidonate from phospholipids. Since MAP kinase activation has been shown to positively regulate cPLA2 activation, data showing that a selective p44/p42 MAPK inhibitor attenuated sPLA2-induced arachidonate production was consistent with this idea. This mechanism provides a plausible explanation as to why adding sPLA2, which catalytically is not selective for arachidonate-containing phospholipids, selectively releases arachidonate and not oleate or linoleate from mast cells. It is known that cPLA2 selectively hydrolyzes arachidonate-containing phospholipids.

Cell adhesion molecules and leukocyte trafficking

Chairpersons: Denis Schrier (Parke-Davis)
Fandrew Issekutz (Dalhousie University)

A series of excellent workshop sessions was organized by James Winkler (Smith-Kline Beecham) and Ken Tramposch (Bristol-Myers Squibb). In the one on "Cell adhesion molecules and leukocyte trafficking", co-chaired by Andrew Issekutz (Dalhousie University, Halifax, Canada) and Denis Schrier (Parke-Davis, Ann Arbor, Michigan), Mike Willwand of Philadelphia College of Osteopathic Medicine (Philadelphia, Pennsylvania) presented an interesting study regarding the induction of CD43 (Leukosialin, Sialophorin) by IL-1. A DNA expression array was differentially probed with reverse transcribed mRNA from synovial fibroblasts stimulated with IL-1 at various time points. At 3 h, both ICAM-1 and CD43 were upregulated. Immunohistochemical analysis of synovial and gingival fibroblasts after IL-1 treatment gave similar results. CD 43 protein was upregulated in a temporal and dose-dependent manner. These findings may indicate an additional means by which blood derived cells adhere to fibroblasts and initiate and/or perpetuate the inflammatory response in inflammatory processes.

Vladimir Vexler of Protein Design Labs (Mountain View, California) described the role of selectins in a rabbit model of LPS-induced subcutaneous inflammation. LPS was injected i.d (100 ng/site) to rabbits on multiple time points before euthanizing the animals at 24 h. The time-course of L-selectin staining on granulocytes, and E- and P-selectin staining on endothelium was evaluated. Simultaneous blockade of all three selectins resulted in a significant decrease in neutrophil counts in histological skin sections and in myeloperoxidase activity in snap frozen skin at early but not late time points. Blockade of selectins individually or the combination of E and P selectin had no effect on neutrophil accumulation. These results suggest that a combination of selectins are involved in leukocyte recruitment and the participation of these molecules is time-dependent.

Gordon Tudderud of Bristol-Myers Squibb (Princeton, New Jersey) presented the profile of an interesting inhibitor of selectin-dependent cell adhesion, BMS-184000(2S,3R4E)-2-hexadecanoylamino-3-benzoyloxy-1-[2,3-di-O-benzoyl-4,6-di-O-(sodium oxysulfonyl)-D-galactopyranosyloxy]-4-octadecene; a synthetic analog of sulfatide). The compound inhibits adhesion of various cell types to P-, E-, and L-

Inflammatory Processes: Molecular Mechanisms and Therapeutic Opportunities, edited by L. Gordon Letts and Douglas W. Morgan

selectin. The compound is active in the acute reverse passive Arthus model in rats and a murine delayed hypersensitivity model. However, the compound had no effect on the onset, frequency or clinical score in murine collagen arthritis, a chronic inflammatory reaction.

In another selectin related presentation, Andrew Issekutz of Dalhousie University (Halifax, Canada) described the role of selectins in eosinphil recruitment in an allergic (ovalbumin, OA) model of lung inflammation in the Brown Norway rat. Adhesion function-blocking monoclonal antibodies to rat P (RMP-1)-, E (RME-1)- and L-selectins (HRL-3 FAB2) were administered in various combinations to the rats and lung eosinophils were quantified in the lung parenchyma and BAL fluid. Treatment with anti-L selectin reduced eosinophils very significantly in the lung. Antibodies to P- or E-selectin did not attenuate the eosinophil accumulation, although dermal inflammation was blocked by these mAbs. Moreover, combination of the anti-P and E-selectin, with anti-L-selectin mAbs did not enhance the inhibition by anti-L selectin administered alone. These results indicate that eosinophil migration to the lungs of OA challenged rats is partially L-selectin dependent. E- and P- selectin appear to contribute little to this process in the lung.

After the break, C.J. DeHaas of Zenica Pharmaceuticals (Wilmington, Delaware) presented an interesting new model for studying human neutrophil migration into lungs of mice challenged with endotoxin by aerosol. Fluorescein labelled human neutrophils were found to migrate into the bronchoalveolar lavage (BAL) fluid within 24 h, with approximately four-fold greater numbers in LPS than in control mice. MAb to human CD18 or CD11b virtually abolished migration into BAL and blockade of mouse ICAM-1 was partially inhibitory. Fucoidin treatment to block selectins was also inhibitory and impressive inhibition was observed with the human neutrophil elastase inhibitors, ICI200880 or ZD8321. A lively discussion followed pointing out the unique features of this model and the interpretation of the findings, given the possibility that human neutrophils may sequester in the mouse lung due to species differences. Nevertheless, the observation that the fluorescent tagged human cells migrated into the BAL, may provide a new approach to study human leukocyte migration in a biological system.

Dr. L.H. Faccioli of the School of Pharmacy of the University of São Paulo (Brazil) presented their group's interesting studies on Mac-1 expression on neutrophils and eosinophils recruited to the peritoneum of mice by i.p. injection of *Histoplasma capsulatum* organisms and the β-glucan containing the F1 cell wall fraction. The recruited neutrophils and eosinophils showed decreased surface expression of Mac-1, especially at time points later than 4 h after initiation of inflammation. This may be a primary effect of the fungus and its products, resulting in inhibition of leukocyte recruitment. However, a secondary effect on leukocyte Mac-1 expression may be due to Mac-1 binding by β-glucan or phagocytosis of particles with endocytosis of the receptor. These possible mechanisms are being investigated. The final paper in the oral presentations was presented by Dr. A. Aruffo of

Bristol Myers Squibb Research Institute (Princeton, New Jersey). He reported the further characterization by this group of the interaction between the Scavenger Receptor Cystine Rich domain (SRCR domain) of CD6 and its interaction with the NH2-terminal immunoglobulin domain of ALCAM, also known as activated leukocyte cell adhesion molecule. CD6 is expressed predominantly on immature and mature T cells and is composed of three SRCR domains and binds to ALCAM (CD166), a member of the immunoglobulin supergene family with 5 Ig like domains. ALCAM is expressed on thymus epithelium and on brain in the human and it is homologous with a neural adhesion molecule in the chicken, believed to be involved in neural guidance. Using site directed mutagenesis, Dr. Aruffo and colleagues characterized the CD6-ALCAM binding, demonstrating that the NH2-terminal first domain of ALCAM binds to domain 3 of CD6. These domains and the binding face are strongly conserved, explaining the cross-species binding observed in this receptor-ligand system. This region of ALCAM, and of other members of the immunoglobulin superfamily, appear to be versatile in mediating interactions with different ligands, broadening opportunities for cell adhesion molecule interactions, some of which may not yet be appreciated.

With this presentation, the adhesion molecule workshop session moved to presentation of three posters the next day. These included an interesting poster by E. Solito et al. from Institute Cochin de Genetique Moleculaire (Paris, France) demonstrating inhibition by Annexin 1 of monocyte adhesion to brain endothelium. This group demonstrated that recombinant Annexin 1 co-localized with VLA-4 on U937 monoblasts, but not with LFA-1 and resulted in inhibition of adhesion to TNF activated human brain endothelium. This raises the possibility that Annexin 1 may modulate adhesion molecule function as one of the effects of glucorticoids. L. Bian of the Department of Ophthalmology and Visual Sciences (Louisville, Kentucky) reported their findings on microvascular endothelial cells harvested from the ciliary process. They demonstrated induction of ICAM-1 and E-selectin expression by TNF on endothelium from this tissue, a structure that not infrequently is involved in systemic vaculitides and autoimmune conditions. Finally, L.H. Faccioli of the School of Pharmacy of University of São Paulo (Brazil) reported on adhesion molecule expression during the acute inflammatory response to *M. tuberculosis* in the mouse peritoneal cavity. Expression of VLA-4 and Mac-1 was diminished on exudate cells compared to cells harvested from uninfected animals. These adhesion receptors may have been down-regulated by the *M. tuberculosis* exposure and may be one mechanism of host immune evasion by this pathogen.

At the workshop presentations and posters, there was fruitful and lively discussion. Important new information was presented, which demonstrates that this continues to be a very active and productive area of research. We are grateful to the Inflammation Research Association and the organizers, especially James Winkler and Kenneth Tramposch for convening this workshop and helping provide this opportunity for scientific exchange.

Pulmonary inflammation, fibrosis, and disease

Chairpersons: Robert M. Strieter (University of Michigan)
David Underwood (SmithKline Beecham)

Inflammation constitutes the host's response to a variety of insults, including trauma, infection, multiorgan failure associated with sepsis, cancer, allograft rejection, ischemia-reperfusion injury, and immunologically mediated processes. Historically the lung has been perceived as an organ primarily involved in gas exchange. However, the lung is an organ anatomically situated interposed between the host and its environment. This barrier consists of not only the airway with its mucociliary clearance, but also the extensive alveolar-capillary wall that is composed of both immune and non-immune cells constantly exposed to both inhaled and hematogenous challenges. Since the lung must maintain its structural integrity for gas exchange, the pulmonary response to these inflammatory stimuli ultimately impacts on host morbidity and mortality.

In the session on "Pulmonary inflammation, fibrosis, and disease", the presentations focused on mechanisms of airway reactivity and inflammation. Airway reactivity and inflammation has been linked to nociceptor tachykinergic mechanisms. Kusner and associates demonstrated that neurokinin receptor antagonism is important in attenuating airway responsiveness. Using a model of guinea pig airway reactivity based on time to onset of dyspnea, these investigators found that the NK2 receptor antagonist ZD7944 was a potent inhibitor of the NK2 receptor agonist (BANK)-induced airway reactivity, but not the airway reactivity associated with the NK1 receptor agonist (ASMSP). In another study, Lengel and associates hypothesized that gastroesophageal reflux-induced airway reactivity is mediated, in part, by tachykinergic mechanisms. To test this postulate, these investigators used an animal model to instill acid into the esophagus and determined whether neurokinin receptor antagonism would attenuate the associated increase in airway inflammation and reactivity. The selective NK1 receptor antagonist (SR140333) abolished the increase in airway mucosal vascular permeability, but did not inhibit airway reactivity. In contrast, the selective NK2 receptor antagonist (ZM274773) attenuated the increase in airway reactivity in response to instillation of esophageal acid. These results suggested that changes in airway inflammation and reactivity in response to gastroesophageal reflux are due to activation of both receptors, and NK1 antago-

Inflammatory Processes: Molecular Mechanisms and Therapeutic Opportunities, edited by L. Gordon Letts and Douglas W. Morgan
© 2000 Birkhäuser Verlag Basel/Switzerland

nism is associated with inhibition of inflammation, whereas, NK2 antagonism is associated with attenuation of airway reactivity. While this study demonstrated the importance of both NK1 and NK2 receptors in mediating airway reactivity and inflammation in response to noxious stimulus, Greenfeder and colleagues, using a strategy of site-directed mutagenesis, determined that a novel non-peptide dual antagonist of NK1 and NK2 receptors, structurally based on MDL 103,392, could mediate its effects *via* distinct binding sites on the NK1 and NK2 receptors. These studies suggested that NK1 and NK2 receptor antagonism may represent a novel therapeutic approach to the treatment of asthma.

The inflammatory response associated with leukocyte infiltration is a salient feature of asthma. Mechanisms of leukocyte recruitment into the airway under conditions of airway reactivity have not been fully elucidated. To determine whether leukotriene antagonism is important to attenuate the inflammatory response associated with allergen challenge, Blain and associates examined the effect of peptidoleukotriene antagonism in a murine model of allergic asthma. They found that administration of the selective LTD4 antagonist, MK-571, alone or in conjunction with the glucocorticoid, dexamethasone, was an effective means to block allergen-induced airway reactivity, vascular permeability, and infiltration of eosinophils. To further examine the importance of the interaction of glucocorticoids with other mediators of inflammation during allergen-induced airway inflammation and reactivity, Kung and associates examined the effect of adrenalectomy on the inhibitory activity of the phosphodiesterase isozyme 4 inhibitor, rolipram. While rolipram treatment blocked airway reactivity and eosinophil airway infiltration, adrenalectomy of these animals markedly attenuated the effect of rolipram on inhibiting the parameters of airway inflammation and reactivity during allergen challenge. These results suggest that adrenal-derived factors (i.e. glucocorticoids and catecholamines) add to the inhibitory effects of rolipram. To further examine whether leukocyte adhesion molecule expression is a contributing factor to leukocyte extravasation during allergen challenge, Richard and associates demonstrated that a small molecule CS-1 peptidomimetic VLA-4 (CD49d) antagonist, CY-9701, could significantly inhibit airway inflammation in allergen challenged mice. In animals challenged with ovalbumin, the VLA-4 antagonist, CY-9701, administered intranasal markedly attenuated both total cellular influx and eosinophilia in bronchoalveolar lavage (BAL) specimens. In addition, inhibition of leukocyte infiltration was associated with a significant reduction in the BAL levels of both IL-4 and IL-5. These findings suggest that inhibition of CD49d ligand-receptor interaction may be an important strategy to block the infiltration of specific leukocytes that play an important role in mediating airway inflammation associated with asthma. Finally, in a non-human primate model of asthma, LaMantia and colleagues demonstrated that *Ascaris suum* challenge induces increased airway responsiveness in *Cynomolgus* monkeys that is associated with the infiltration of neutrophils followed temporally by the influx of eosinophils. The kinetics of leukocyte extravasation in this model system was paralleled by the presence of both CXC and CC chemokines in the BAL of these animals, suggesting that these cytokines may be playing a role in the elicitation of leukocytes during allergen challenge in these animals, and this response may be analogous to what is occurs in human asthma. The above studies exemplify the importance of a variety of mediators that may act alone or in an interactive manner contributing to the pathogenesis of airway reactivity and inflammation. Future studies will further delineate the relative importance of each of these factors in human asthma.

Angiogenesis, wound repair and skin inflammation

Chairpersons: W. Hunter (Angiotech)
E. Turley (Hospital for Sick Children, Toronto)

This session, held on Tuesday evening, Nov. 3, 1998, included in its first half an eclectic mix of reports describing aspects of the biology of angiogenic ligands/receptors *in vitro* and *in vivo*. In the second half of the session, reports focused upon human or models of human psoriasis and molecules that may contribute to this skin disease. The first report entitled "Quantitation of Ang-1 and -2 mRNA in rheumatoid synovial fibroblasts by Taqman™ quantitative PCR" by Scott et al., described a differential effect of pro-inflammatory cytokines/growth factors on the levels of Ang-1, -2 produced by RA synovial fibroblasts. The ability of TGFB and TNFα to upregulate Ang-1 but not -2 mRNA levels suggests a role for this Tie-2 ligand in rheumatoid arthritis. The second report entitled "Stimulation of Tie-2 receptors activates signal transduction through Grb2 and SH-PTP in HuUVECS and stimulates angiogenesis *in vivo*" by Hansbury et al. describes the use of agonist high affinity mAbs to Tie-2 receptor to assess signaling pathways regulated by this receptor. Data show that the mAb promoted receptor phosphorylation and also co-association of the adaptor protein Grb2 as well as SH-PTP as assessed by immunoprecipitation assays. Further, the antibody promoted angiogenesis in mice, indicating a role for the Tie-2 receptor and the above signaling molecules in angiogenesis. The third report entitled "Pharmacological modulation of VEGF expression induced by hypoxia and IL-1β" by Jackson et al. described investigations of the signaling pathways that control VEGF expression, an important angiogenic factor, by hypoxia and by IL-1β. Interestingly, expression does not appear to be regulated by common acute signaling pathways including the various map kinase cascades, or PI-3 kinase, suggesting that novel pathways may be involved in control of this important growth factor.

The second half of this session was begun with a report entitled "Evaluation of topical paclitaxel gel as a potential treatment for psoriasis" by Toleikis et al. describing impressive *in vitro* and *in vivo* results showing the anti-inflammatory and anti-proliferative properties of paclitaxel. Further, this compound was shown to inhibit expression of collagenase and stromelysin by human microvascular endothelial cells *in vitro*. In a mouse model of contact hypersensitivity, paclitaxel gel significantly

Inflammatory Processes: Molecular Mechanisms and Therapeutic Opportunities, edited by L. Gordon Letts and Douglas W. Morgan
© 2000 Birkhäuser Verlag Basel/Switzerland

inhibited ear swelling and erythema suggesting that paclitaxel may be efficaceous in treatment of human psoriasis. The second report entitled "Histological and immunocytochemical evaluation of human psoriasis: implications for a human anti-inflammatory *in vivo* screening model" by Chosay et al., documents the changes in histopathological features, vascularity, adhesion molecules (ICAM-1, PECAM-1), key transcription factor cellular localization and leukocyte infiltration during the evolution of psoriatic skin lesions. Results suggest that psoriatic lesions share many features of other inflammatory processes and human psoriasis may offer a tractable model for rapid screening of anti-inflammatory reagents. The final report entitled "Brp-39 and YM-1 are differentially upregulated in murine models of skin inflammation" by Tierney et al. describes the expression of two novel proteins belonging to the mammalian chitinase-related glycoprotein family in chronic contact hypersensitivity and acute inflammatory models of the skin. YM-1 was strongly upregulated in hyperplastic epidermis following oxazolone exposure but not UV exposure. In contrast, Brp-39 was moderately upregulated in both models. These results suggest a rather specific role of YM-1 in chronic contact hypersensitivity.

This session was well attended and produced active discussion of the interesting presentations.

Index